Praise for *The Smart Woman's Guide to Diabetes*

"…we can't think of a better researched guide to the nuanced life of a woman with diabetes than Amy Stockwell Mercer's new book *The Smart Woman's Guide to Diabetes.*"

—DiabetesMine

"This is not a very large book, but I was surprised how complete and comprehensive it is. It feels as if you are chatting with a group of friends who truly understand what it is like to live as a woman with diabetes and it does not get boring or become a chore to read. I highly recommend this one."

—Elizabeth Woolley, about.com Type 2 Diabetes Guide

"Imparting critical information for diabetic women in pursuit of a healthy and fulfilling life, Mercer covers a range of topics, including finding the right medical team, gaining control through information and communication, managing adolescence, diet, and exercise. Special attention is given to eating disorders and body image; dating, sex, and marriage; pregnancy and motherhood; and telling others about one's condition. An excellent resource for those seeking information about the impact of diabetes on women's lives; the many personal stories lend warmth and accessibility."

—Library Journal

"Well worth a look, it presents a wide variety of experiences, viewpoints, and approaches to diabetes management. This is the greatest strength of this book, making it of most use to recently diagnosed women (whatever stage of life they may be) who are trying to navigate unfamiliar thoughts, feelings, and concerns about themselves, their health, and their safety."

—Emily Coles, tudiabetes

"Amy Stockwell Mercer calls her new book, *The Smart Woman's Guide to Diabetes*, a labor of love. It covers aspects of women's lives ranging from eating to dating to raising children, all while coping with diabetes."

—Diabetes Forecast

"Amy's book covers every aspect of being female and living with diabetes, beginning with a diagnosis at any age. She covers schooling, relationships, exercising, eating, traveling, pregnancy, parenting, menopause, and more. This great guide is packed with solid wisdom, advice, and guidance that will help any woman with this condition live a happier and healthier life."

—Cheryl Alkon, Author of *Balancing Pregnancy With Pre-Existing Diabetes: Healthy Mom, Healthy Baby*

"Having had type 1 diabetes for more than 25 years and having written 2 books on the subject, I enjoyed reading Amy Mercer's book very much. It is well written and covers every aspect of living with diabetes across the life span from a woman's perspective. I especially liked the chapters on diagnosis, pregnancy, travel, and aging gracefully. It is worth reading for women living with diabetes at whatever stage in life they are and for the family and friends who love them."

—Rita G. Mertig, MS, RNC, CNS, DE, Author, What Nurses Know Diabetes and Guide to Teaching Diabetes Self-Management

"...a heaping dose of wisdom for dealing with diabetes on any front of one's life and living well through it all. Dealing with the many potential complications of life with grace and wisdom, *The Smart Woman's Guide to Diabetes* is a thoughtful and useful read for anyone making the most of their lives in spite of diabetes."

—Midwest Book Review

The *Smart Woman's* Guide to Eating Right with Diabetes

The *Smart Woman's* Guide to Eating Right with Diabetes

What Will Work

Amy Stockwell Mercer

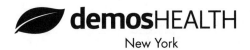

New York

Visit our website at www.demoshealth.com

ISBN: 9781936303373
e-book ISBN: 9781617051241

Acquisitions Editor: Noreen Henson
Compositor: diacriTech

Medical information provided by Demos Health, in the absence of a visit with a health care professional, must be considered as an educational service only. This book is not designed to replace a physician's independent judgment about the appropriateness or risks of a procedure or therapy for a given patient. Our purpose is to provide you with information that will help you make your own health care decisions.

The information and opinions provided here are believed to be accurate and sound, based on the best judgment available to the authors, editors, and publisher, but readers who fail to consult appropriate health authorities assume the risk of injuries. The publisher is not responsible for errors or omissions. The editors and publisher welcome any reader to report to the publisher any discrepancies or inaccuracies noticed.

Library of Congress Cataloging-in-Publication Data

Mercer, Amy.
  The smart woman's guide to eating right with diabetes : what will work /
Amy Stockwell Mercer.
     p. cm.
Includes index.
ISBN 978-1-936303-37-3
  1. Diabetes in women--Popular works. 2. Diabetes--Diet therapy--Popular
works. I. Title.
RC660.4.M466 2013
616.4'620654--dc23
                              2012030116

Special discounts on bulk quantities of Demos Health books are available to corporations, professional associations, pharmaceutical companies, health care organizations, and other qualifying groups. For details, please contact:

Special Sales Department
Demos Medical Publishing, LLC
11 West 42nd Street, 15th Floor
New York, NY 10036
Phone: 800-532-8663 or 212-683-0072
Fax: 212-941-7842
E-mail: rsantana@demosmedpub.com

Printed in the United States of America by Bang Printing.
12 13 14 15 / 5 4 3 2 1

*This book is dedicated to the four men
in my life: my husband Dale,
and my three amazing sons:
Will, Miles, and Reid.*

Contents

Foreword

Diabetes makes a terrible dinner date.

It asks for all the sauces on the side. It second-guesses whatever it just ordered, then it fiddles with a needle or a pump under the table-cloth. Diabetes asks for juice when the salads are delayed. When the salads arrive, diabetes picks out the carrots because carrots have a high glycemic index. Then it chatters on about "the glycemic index" as if that's interesting dinner conversation.

Diabetes skips dessert. Or it has dessert but then feels bad about it all night long. Diabetes' nightcap is a bolus. Its goodnight kiss tastes like a glucose tablet.

I've been taking my diabetes to dinner for eighteen years, since my diagnosis at age twenty-five when I was smack at the beginning of my career and wanting very much to fit in with my colleagues at business lunches and office potlucks. Diabetes was a clumsy companion I wanted to ditch at the door.

The only way I could do that was to pretend I'd already eaten, or pretend that of all the appetizers on the buffet, I truly and only loved plain celery. That kept my diabetes a secret, but after a potluck or two, it made me seem anorexic-ish. Which I probably actually was. Disordered eating is an easy side street down which many of us tiptoe in pursuit of better A1Cs and smoother dinner dates.

Fortunately, there are better strategies. Amy Stockwell Mercer is on to a lot of them. And fortunately, she wants to share them with us, as she did in *The Smart Woman's Guide to Diabetes* and as she does so well online at www.amystockwellmercer.com.

In *The Smart Woman's Guide to Eating Right With Diabetes*, Amy gives us plenty of honest truth from her own experience and from the interviews she's conducted with men and women who have discovered new, surprising, unconventional, and often simple means of eating right. Amy also shares clinical research with clarity and compassion. And through it all, she threads a unique and welcome brand of encouragement.

She is quick to acknowledge that eating right with diabetes is not a lot of fun. Diabetes is not the dinner date any of us imagined, or desired, or necessarily feel like entertaining for the rest of our lives.

But Amy is making the best of it, and she believes we can, too.

So please join us. Have a seat. Order what works, however it works for you.

Ann Rosenquist Fee, MA, MFA
Singer, writer, parent, partner, tarot reader,
smart woman with diabetes
www.annrosenquistfee.com

Preface

When I was diagnosed with diabetes in 1985, I was fourteen years old, and my favorite foods were Cherry Coke, Sugar Babies, and chocolate milkshakes. I was living away from home for the first time in my young life at a boarding high school in New Hampshire. We lived in dorms with dorm parents, and some of us who lived close enough went home on the weekends. My life at home was very different from my life at school, and I sometimes felt like I was being pulled in two different directions.

Mom and Dad were vegetarian hippies who had a garden out back and a kitchen full of whole grains, canned tomatoes, and whole milk with the cream floating on top (for mom's coffee) from the dairy farm down the dirt road, and warm eggs from our chickens who pooped in our old sandbox. Mom and Dad thought that sugar was bad for my sister and me, and had been restricting our intake since the day we were born. Our birthday cakes were made of carob chocolate and our ice cream was churned in a large container with a crank that seemed to require hours of cranking. By the time it was "ready," it was melting and had to be drunk from the bowl with a straw. All of this seemed mostly normal to me until I went away to boarding school.

At Proctor Academy we could go to the "den" after study hall and order Philly cheesesteaks and French fries and chocolate milkshakes and charge it to our personal accounts. The first time I watched a friend say "charge it to my account" at the counter after she'd ordered, I ran back to the dorm to call my parents on the hallway pay phone (1985, remember) and ask why I didn't have a charge account. My parents were borrowing money to send me to this school and didn't budge when I begged and pleaded for a charge account at the den. "You have a great cafeteria where you can eat for free," dad said. I didn't want to go to the cafeteria; I wanted to go to the den with my friends. I also wanted to go to the mini-mart across the street after field hockey practice with my friends to buy Cherry Cokes and Sugar Babies for our post-practice snack, so I learned to save what I could from my monthly allowance. There, I indulged in all the food my parents had forbidden, and I didn't feel guilty because my parents had no idea. I was making up for all those years of carob cookies and fiddleheads. I tried smoking a cigarette, stayed up late listening to the older girls in the dorm talk about sex, and flirted with an older boy. It was six weeks of thrilling freedom, until I got sick.

Being diagnosed with type 1 diabetes felt like the gods were punishing me. Diabetes was a literal wall crashing down on my freedom, and it felt as if my body was rebelling against my wild ways. For a fourteen-year-old girl, diabetes meant rules and restrictions, it meant eating three times a day, it meant giving myself shots when it was time to eat, it meant listening to my body when all I wanted to do was use my body to propel me from one exciting adventure to the next. It meant thinking about food like an adult (carbohydrate counting, nutritional information, reading labels), and it meant thinking about food as medicine.

Diabetes was a lot of work, and I didn't have the time or interest in counting carbohydrates and figuring out how much insulin I needed for what I was eating. When my diabetes educator and nutritionist would ask me about my insulin to carb ratio, I shrugged. My A1Cs were good, so no one bothered me about it. I'd had diabetes for long enough that I acted like I couldn't bother myself with their pesky questions, charts, and numbers. I just ate the same thing at almost every meal and guessed at my insulin needs. If I was high after a meal, I gave another shot, and if I were low, I'd drink a glass of juice. It wasn't ideal, but it worked for me. Besides, I didn't want to be told what to do by someone who didn't have diabetes. They had no idea how hard it was to count everything I ate, so why should I listen to them?

That's why I wanted to write this book as a follow up to *The Smart Woman's Guide to Diabetes*. There are two chapters in that first book that focus on eating, but there is so much more to say. When it comes to eating "right" or "wrong" with diabetes, the opinions and lessons are many. I've lived with diabetes for twenty-six years, and one of the favorite things I like to tell people when I'm speaking at a diabetes event is that I am not an expert. I will never be an expert on diabetes, because diabetes management depends on the individual, and it changes day to day and year to year. What I ate when I was fourteen is not even on my radar now that I am forty-one years old. What worked for me then will not work for me today, and what works for me today might not work in another five years. As women with diabetes we have to be flexible, we have to be patient, and we have to listen to our bodies. We all know this, and we all continue to learn.

For those who look at this book and think, "What does she know about eating right with diabetes?" I'll answer that what I know is what I've learned from the women I've interviewed for this book. I wrote this book because I wanted to answer my questions about eating right with diabetes. I wanted to understand why my blood sugar was often high first thing in the morning and why I was sometimes starving when I'd just finished a meal. I knew I wasn't the only one with these questions. I also knew that I preferred to get my answers from other women with diabetes—women who live with diabetes, women like you and me. Some of these women are experts in the field of eating right and others are regular women like you and me who've worked hard to determine what works for them when it comes to eating right. I am not an expert, but I've learned a lot while researching and writing this book.

In these pages you will read the collected stories from interviews with people living with diabetes, type 1 and type 2, as well as experts in the field of nutrition. The stories are wide ranging and offer a glimpse into a variety of diets, from low carbohydrate to vegetarianism to raw foods and the standard American diet. It is my belief that there is no "one size fits all" when it comes to eating right, and that what works for me as a forty-one-year-old mom, may not work for a college freshman. The book is divided into chapters, so you can read the sections and "diets" that interest you and hear stories from individuals who have found success with these diets. And I'm using the term "diet" for clarity's sake only. I have never liked the word diet because I'm not trying to lose weight— I'm trying to eat well and live a healthy life, and that word comes with a lot of baggage. I'm going to try to stay away from the term diet and use "healthy eating plans," because I think part of the problem with eating right for so many Americans has to do with the word diet. Diet is about numbers: pounds gained and pounds lost, or phrases like: I went off my diet, I'm back on my diet, I'm on a roller-coaster diet, I'm a yo-yo dieter. I think in order to change our way of thinking about food and Eating Right, we need to talk of and treat food as a source of nourishment, a way to care for our families and ourselves, a way for people with diabetes to fuel our bodies.

After twenty-six years of living with diabetes, I think I'm beginning to figure out how to "eat right." It took many years of disordered eating behaviors before I changed my way of thinking about and eating food, and while I'm proud to say that today I'm living well with diabetes, it will always require effort. In these pages, I hope you will find inspiration, tips, and advice on how to nourish and fuel your body with food.

Acknowledgments

This book was built by a team of amazing women who shared their personal and private stories with me about life with diabetes. Thank you: Ann Rosenquist Fee, Ana Morales, Aliza Chana Zaelon, Alyssa Rosenzweig, Brandy Barnes, Cheryl Alkon, Ginger Vieira, Heather Nielsen Clute, Katie Peterson, Kelly Love Johnson, Lesley Hoffman Goldenberg, Linda Frick, Michelle Sorensen, Rachel Garlinghouse, and Sysy Morales.

Thanks to the doctors, endocrinologists, nutritionists, and diabetes educators who have helped me to live well with diabetes. I'd also like to give a special shout out to Franziska Spritzler, RD, CDE, who is quoted throughout this book and graciously shared her advice during the final edits of the manuscript.

This book is written by women living with diabetes, not by medical professionals.

The opinions expressed are a reflection of the experiences of the author and the women interviewed as they have sought to find eating plans that work for them. If you are interested in adopting an eating plan that is outlined in this book, please consult with your personal nutritionist and other health care professionals.

1

History of Diabetes: "The Starvation Diet"

When I was first diagnosed in 1985, the nurse told me that when I was hungry between meals, I could snack on "free foods."

"What are free foods?" I asked, thinking she meant food that didn't cost any money.

"Free foods are foods you can eat without having to give a shot, foods that are low in carbohydrates such as nuts and pickles," she beamed at me. I hated nuts and I hated pickles.

"Can I still drink Cherry Coke?" I asked, not looking at my mother who didn't know that while I was away at school, I'd developed a love of Cherry Coke. (Cherry Coke was a brand new flavor in 1985. Diet Cherry Coke was not introduced until the following year.)

"No, Cherry Coke has a lot of sugar. You can drink water or tea," the nurse said in all seriousness.

"Tea?" I looked at my mother. Tea was something grandmothers drank. Tea was something you had with honey and a lemon when you were sick. This nurse wanted me to trade Cherry Coke for tea? Mom smiled and reached over to rub my shoulder. I wanted to scream.

That first year may have been one of the hardest. One week I was a healthy fourteen-year-old, and the next I was a young woman with a chronic illness. I had to re-learn how to eat. Food became an ongoing lesson in science and biology, subjects that often seemed over my head. All I knew in those first few months was that I could no longer eat my favorite foods and that made me frustrated and sad.

I learned many years later that the history of diabetes began not with "free foods" but with starvation. As early as the sixteenth century, starvation was used as a treatment for diabetes. Starving a patient meant removing food from someone who was complaining of frequent urination, unquenchable thirst, and endless fatigue. It was a desperate act used as a last resort.

I remember these sensations. At fourteen years old I remember feeling so thirsty that I was dreaming about water. I remember being so tired that I couldn't keep my eyes open in French class. I remember being hungry, too, a hunger that physically hurt, a hunger that seemed insatiable, a hunger that didn't make sense because I was losing so much weight that I could see the outline of my ribs when I lifted up my shirt. I remember sitting on my bed in my room, drinking a strawberry milkshake, and falling back onto my pillow in defeat. I was too tired, too thirsty, and too hungry to get up. I didn't know what was wrong with me, and I was afraid to ask. When I finally did ask for help, the nurse at school thought I was starving myself on purpose because I'd lost so much weight. I was soon diagnosed with type 1 diabetes in 1985, given insulin, and my hunger and thirst disappeared. It's been twenty-six years since that day and when I look back on the history of diabetes, I can't imagine being as sick as I was and hearing that the only way to keep me alive was to go without.

By 1913, the starvation diet was still the only method to keep patients alive. Dr. Frederick Allen, a researcher of sugar consumption at Harvard Medical School was placing his weakened, dehydrated, and ill patients on a fast until the sugar was gone from their body. This fast typically took a few days, and when the sugar was gone from their urine, small amounts of food such as vegetables boiled three times (to decrease their carbohydrate content), butter, and bacon were slowly added to their diets. The typical diet consisted of 800 to 1,000 calories per day, and patients were carefully monitored. If sugar was detected in their urine, the diet was dropped back to the previous day's measurements. Dr. Allen's patients had been brought to him because there simply was no other option.

The starvation diet was not sustainable and required close supervision and monitoring. Difficult to maintain, this diet often made the patient's last few months of life miserable. In "Why Were 'Starvation Diets' Promoted for Diabetes in the Pre-Insulin Period?"

(*Nutrition Journal*), Allan Mazur writes that looking back on this time Dr. Elliott Joslin, the founder of the Joslin Diabetes Center, said, *"We literally starved the child and adult with the faint hope that something new in treatment would appear ... It was no fun to starve a child to let him live.'"*

One of Dr. Allen's first patients was a blind twelve-year-old boy already in bad shape when first seen in 1914, seven years after onset. Mazur writes that Dr. Allen experimented with various diets and periods of fasting and was puzzled by unaccountable glucose found in the boy's urine, unrelated to the known food intake.

Allen remarks in his write-up, "It seemed that a blind boy isolated in a hospital room and so weak that he could scarcely leave his bed would not be able to obtain food surreptitiously when only trustworthy persons were admitted. It turned out that his supposed helplessness was the very thing that gave him opportunities that other persons lacked. ... Among the unusual things eaten were tooth-paste and bird-seed, the latter being obtained from the cage of a canary which he had asked for. Also his mother and his governess on visiting him sometimes brought lunch, which was kept in a closet, supposedly without his knowledge; nonetheless, in the short intervals when he was unwatched, he managed to find it and remove such articles as might not be missed. These facts were obtained by confession after long and plausible denials." This boy died after four months of treatment.

Dr. Allen saw calorie restriction as the reason for successful cases, and lapses from diet as the reason for failures. The language used to describe this sick child's condition "Obtain[ing] food surreptitiously," and "confession" and "denials," built the foundation of a diabetic diet. How many of us today, almost one hundred years later, feel like we are "sneaking" or "cheating" when it comes to food? How many of us think we've done something "bad" when our blood sugars are high or low after a meal? Perhaps these attitudes exist because of the history of diabetes?

The history of our nation, the history of our people, our forefathers, of all those who came before us, created the foundation we stand on today. We look to the past in order to learn how to improve on or to repeat the things we deem important. History reminds us of who we are, where we've been, and where we are going. Therefore, it seems reasonable to suggest that the history of diabetes has shaped our attitude toward food today. It's my belief that people with diabetes have a win-or-lose attitude toward food because the treatment for diabetes began with starvation.

Dr. Joslin came on the scene in 1915 and adopted Allen's treatment, first removing fat, then protein, then carbohydrate from the diet, forestalling hyperglycemic crises and ketoacidosis that can induce diabetic coma. In the 1920s, insulin was discovered and everything changed. People with diabetes could eat again, and over the years management became about measuring food-to-insulin intake. Dr. Joslin continued to work tirelessly for years helping people manage their diabetes, espousing the long-term benefits of tight blood sugar control, and in the 1990s the Diabetes Control and Complications Trial (DCCT), a landmark medical study conducted by the United States National Institute of Diabetes and Digestive and Kidney Diseases (NIDDK), verified Joslin's position and showed tight blood sugar control reduced diabetes complications.

Today there are approximately thirty million people with diabetes in the United States and another eighty million with pre-diabetes, and almost as many different opinions on how to eat right with diabetes, There is still no one size fits all when it comes to eating right with diabetes so it's no wonder we get confused when it comes time to eat. I've lived with diabetes for twenty-six years and continue to learn something new every day about eating right. Some of the best advice I've learned has come from other men and women living with diabetes, and their stories will be shared with readers in these pages. I'm thankful that our methods for managing blood sugars have improved, which in turn have created a wider variety of eating options. We have come a long way in my personal history with diabetes and even further in the history of diabetes.

FOOD MYTHS

Myths about diabetes are both frustrating and embarrassing. Everyone has heard them and everyone has a different approach when it comes to responding to the myth. What is your approach? Do you get defensive or do you use the myth as an opportunity to educate the public about living with diabetes?

Michelle Sorensen was diagnosed with type 1 diabetes a few weeks before her twenty-fifth birthday. She has now lived with this disease for twelve years. "Sometimes the general myths about diabetes, not just food related ones, still have the ability to rattle me. Something came up recently about my diabetes with a neighbor who is my age, with young kids. She is kind of outspoken and not always the most sensitive. All the same, when she said: 'Hey, don't people with diabetes have bad breath?' I was kind of stunned. Of course, there is a kernel of truth in that those with uncontrolled sugars can have 'sweet' breath, but even if I fit that category, I wasn't sure how that question would be okay to ask. I don't even remember how I responded but it made me feel the way I did in the first few years I had diabetes ... like it was a dirty secret I shouldn't tell people. I wonder how many people have those kinds of stereotypes about diabetes."

Myth #1   People with Diabetes Have to Eat Different Foods from the Rest of the Family

People with diabetes can eat the same foods as the rest of their family. Current nutrition guidelines for diabetes are very flexible and offer many choices, allowing people with diabetes to fit in favorite or special-occasion foods. Everyone, whether they have diabetes or not, should eat a healthful diet that consists of fruits, vegetables, whole grains, lean protein foods, and heart-healthy fats. So, if you have diabetes, there's no need to cook separately from your family.

Riva Greenberg, author of *50 Diabetes Myths That Can Ruin Your Life: And The 50 Diabetes Truths That Can Save It*, says she never eats anything specially made for diabetics. "Sugar-free and diabetic foods often have as many calories, carbs, and fats as regular foods. There's no need to buy anything that says 'Made for diabetics.' If I want something sweet I eat the real thing, whether it's a peanut butter cookie or slice of pumpkin pie. I just eat less of it—like half a serving—and not on a regular basis. Recently I was in Southern California visiting my cousin. She picked me up at the airport and as we were driving to her house I said, 'Let's stop for an ice cream cone.' She said, 'You said that to me the last time you were here!' I said, 'It's probably the last time I had one!' and she said, 'No wonder you never gain weight!'"

Rachel Garlinghouse agrees and says, "I have been told how great sugar-free products are for diabetics. But sugar-free doesn't mean carb-free, and many 'sugar-free' products are laden with other bad-for-you ingredients like food dyes, transfats, hydrogenated oils, and more. Additionally, many artificial sweeteners can cause gastric issues in their consumers. There have been studies linking artificial sweeteners to other issues, including cancer; however, many believe these studies are unfounded. I think sugar-free products and products containing artificial sweeteners taste terrible; therefore, I don't consume them. And some studies have shown that people who consume artificial sugars tend to weigh more than those who consume regular sugar. It is believed by some that the body knows when sugars are fake and it craves more sugar, so those who consume artificial sugars tend to overeat over the course of the day, trying to satisfy their body's cravings. Instead of consuming any artificial sugars, I reduce the amount of sugar in my baking recipes and use higher-fiber and higher-protein ingredients to improve the nutritional value of the foods I make. Additionally, I eat as much organic food as possible, plenty of produce, and I have chosen a vegetarian diet. Almost all of my family's meals are homemade so I know exactly what is in the foods I'm consuming."

Myth #2   People with Diabetes Should Never Give in to Food Cravings

Almost everyone has food cravings at some point, and people with diabetes are no exception. It's not uncommon for people with diabetes to cut out all sweets or even cut way back on food portions in order to lose weight. In turn, your body often responds to these drastic changes by creating cravings. Nine times out of ten, your food choices in these situations tend to be high in fat and/or sugar, too.

The best way to deal with food cravings is to try to prevent them by following a healthy eating plan that lets you occasionally fit sweets into your diabetes meal plan. If a craving does occur, let yourself have a small taste of whatever it is you want. By doing so, you can enjoy the flavor and avoid overeating later on.

Linda Frick was diagnosed in 1961, or as she calls it, "the dark ages of diabetes care," and says she remembers the nurse at the hospital telling her she could never eat ice cream again. "That was my first introduction to diabetes and I cried," she says. "I can remember a few years back during the holidays I was at Costco with my daughter and they were giving out free samples of different food products. There was a booth with something sweet, and my daughter asked the person behind the table if they made them sugar free as I reached for one to try. Since I'm on the pump, I can occasionally eat limited quantities of sweet things, however when the person behind the table found out I was diabetic, she literally yelled across the store that I couldn't have that sample. I tried to explain but she wasn't listening. It was uncomfortable. After fifty years of this I should be used to it. It's frustrating."

Myth #3   People with Diabetes Shouldn't Eat Too Many Starchy Foods, Even if They Contain Fiber, because Starch Raises Your Blood Glucose and Makes You Gain Weight

Starchy foods, such as bread, pasta, rice, and cereal, provide carbohydrate, the body's primary energy source. Fruit, milk, yogurt, and desserts contain carbohydrate as well. Everyone needs some carbohydrate in their diet, even people with diabetes. Weight gain occurs when you take in more calories than you burn off. So, if you eat too much of *any* food, you'll end up gaining weight. The key is knowing how much to eat of all the good food groups to help keep blood glucose levels in a safe range and keep you at a healthy weight. Choose starchy foods that are whole grain and high in fiber for overall good nutrition.

Ann Rosenquist Fee was diagnosed when she was trying to get pregnant with her first child. Of the power of myths she says, "Early in my first year with diabetes, I realized that fifteen carbs of apple wasn't the same as fifteen carbs of orange juice or cake or Cheerios. Cheerios were about the worst. They led to my highest postprandials. When I'd take more Novolog the next time to try to cover the same amount, my numbers might be better an hour later but I'd be down in the fifties quickly after that.

"I told my dietitian about it and asked if we should maybe change my meal plan to be mostly fruit and hardly any refined starches. Not that I wanted to quit Cheerios. I really didn't. But I really hated seeing so many highs and I was running out of ideas for how to keep them under control.

"My dietitian said it wasn't a good idea. She said the ADA [American Diabetes Association] said fifteen carbs was fifteen carbs, and the USDA said I needed several servings of starch every day. Up to that point, I'd done everything she'd told me to do. I'd weighed all my food, tracked what I ate, and ate just how the pyramid said. After the apple/Cheerios talk, I followed some of her advice but treated the rest as myth—fine ideas but not necessarily true for me. I still listen to what dietitians and the ADA and USDA have to say, but I give my body the last word. And the last word on Cheerios is (usually) no."

Myth #4   People with Diabetes Do Not Have to Worry about Eating Fat Because It Doesn't Have Much of an Effect on Blood Glucose

Fat, found in margarine, oils, and salad dressings, has little immediate effect on blood glucose levels. However, eating a fatty meal can slow down digestion and make it harder for your insulin to work, causing a possible high blood glucose level hours after your meal. Some fats can raise blood cholesterol, increasing your risk for heart attack or stroke. These fats are called saturated fat and trans fat and should be limited as much as possible. Sources of saturated fat include: butter, red meat, cheese, and whole milk. Trans fat is found in shortening, some margarines, snack foods, and fast foods. Also, fat is very high in calories and should be limited if you're trying to lose weight.

Myth #5   Eating Too Much Sugar Causes Diabetes

The causes of diabetes are still unknown. Family history, a weakened immune system, a virus, and environmental factors are some of the probable causes of type 1 diabetes. Type 2 diabetes is caused by genetics and lifestyle factors. Being overweight does increase your risk for developing type 2 diabetes, and a diet high in calories, whether from sugar or from fat, can contribute to weight gain. If you have a history of diabetes in your family, a healthy meal plan and regular exercise are recommended to manage your weight.

Meagan Esler has lived with type 1 diabetes for over seventeen years and says, "While I'm pretty sure the biggest diabetes food myth of all is that diabetics cannot have sugar, people seem to form many versions of this belief. I've had people I barely know slap my hand over candy, holler over baked goods, overreact to a small bag of potato chips, and even question a simple sandwich. Seems no matter what I eat, people judge.

I often find myself wondering what the diabetes police would have us eat if they were in charge. Of course I shouldn't eat a bunch of cookies, but should anyone? Moderation is a key factor for everyone, not just diabetics. Many people without diabetes don't understand that even a salad can raise our blood sugar significantly if it contains croutons and a sweet dressing. We have to rely on carbohydrate counts and medication dosages to allow for each meal, even the healthiest ones. The caution a person with diabetes must exercise when eating is certainly not limited to chocolate and pastries.

With close to eighteen years of living with diabetes, I've realized that what I eat should be kept between me and my doctor, it's not for the general population to decide. I will not be ashamed of my food choices, I work hard every day to maintain a healthy body and believe that we all deserve a little treat now and then."

Myth #6   You Have to Give Up All Your Favorite Foods When You're on a Diabetes Diet

There is no reason to give up your favorite foods on a diabetes diet. Instead, try:

- Changing the way your favorite foods are prepared.
- Changing the other foods you usually eat along with your favorite foods.
- Reducing the serving sizes of your favorite foods.
- Using your favorite foods as a reward for following your meal plans.

A dietitian can help you find ways to include your favorites in your diabetes meal plans.

Riva Greenberg says, "The typical myth: You can't eat sugar. I remember being told this when I was first diagnosed thirty-nine years ago. Being told I couldn't eat anything with sugar like a candy bar or piece of cake. Of course no one said I shouldn't eat those huge tuna subs on study night in college that had a smear of tuna sitting on a massive loaf of bread roll. That must have shot my blood sugar through the roof! I tried not eating sweets but I'm sure I wasn't entirely successful. Today we know you can eat anything if you balance it with activity and medicine, and that starchy foods like bread, potatoes and rice break down into sugar in your bloodstream just like cookies! Today I don't eat a lot of sweets. I've changed my diet to healthy foods over the years and my tastebuds have changed with it. When I taste typical processed sweets: cookies, candy, cake, pie, they taste much too sweet, artificial and/or greasy. My guilty pleasures are high quality dark chocolate. I'll have a square or two of 85 percent chocolate in the evening when I want something sweet or a sliver of whatever I'm currently addicted to like halvah or gingerbread. As for refined carbs, I basically don't eat them. I've grown to prefer the nutty taste of complex carbohydrates like beans, quinoa, brown rice and sweet potatoes. Yum!"

Myth #7   Carbohydrates Are Bad for Diabetics

Carbohydrates (carbs) form the foundation of a healthy diet. Carbohydrates have the greatest effect on blood sugar levels, which is why you are asked to monitor how many carbohydrates you eat when following a diabetes diet. However, carbohydrate foods contain many essential nutrients, including vitamins, minerals, and fiber. So one diabetes diet tip is to choose those with the most nutrients, like whole-grain breads and baked goods, and high-fiber fruits and vegetables. You may find it easier to select the "best" carbs if you meet with a dietitian.

Alyssa Rosenzweig was diagnosed with type 1 diabetes at ten years old and soon after, discovered she suffered from digestion issues. She says, "I really don't know any other way of eating/exercising/living than my own, but I realized the other day how odd it would be to a nondiabetic to have to count and watch and monitor every bite/move; it's so unnatural. Who would think to take for granted the core function of the body to eat/digest? It's usually an, 'I'm hungry, let's eat' without a passing thought. Or 'I'm too busy to worry about food.' I remember how shocked I was hearing a colleague forget his lunch and how traumatic it would be for me to forget to pack food to eat. I would never do that because I simply wouldn't have anything to eat, there aren't any easy plan-B options. Very little is done on a whim—food and otherwise—which, on a related note about my own character and values, actually makes me love spontaneous moments even more." Alyssa says there is "safety in boring eating" and that she has become well versed in nutrition. "Knowing the difference between 15 grams of carbs from Lucky Charms and 15 grams of carbs from an apple is empowering." Another part of this nontruth that bothers Alyssa is the dessert myth. "When it's my birthday people at work will ask what I want to do to celebrate my birthday and then they'll say, 'Oh but you can't have cake!'" She says, "I don't even like cake." Which brings us to …

Myth #8   You Can't Eat Dessert if You Have Diabetes

Not true! You can develop many strategies for including desserts in a diabetes diet. Here are some examples:

- Use artificial sweeteners in desserts.
- Cut back on the amount of dessert. For example, instead of two scoops of ice cream, have one. Or share a dessert with a friend.
- Use desserts as an occasional reward for following your diabetes diet plan.
- Make desserts more nutritious. For example, use whole grains, fresh fruit, and vegetable oil when preparing desserts. Many times, you can use less sugar than a recipe calls for without sacrificing taste or consistency.
- Expand your dessert horizons. Instead of ice cream, pie, or cake, try fruit, a whole-wheat oatmeal-raisin cookie, (dark) chocolate, or yogurt with nuts.

Megrette Fletcher (Hammond), MEd, RD, CDE, is a registered dietitian, certified diabetes educator, author, and co-founder of The Center for Mindful Eating, says her favorite myth is the "we can't eat" myth. "My personal favorite revolves around the vegetable beets. 'I can't eat beets' or, 'We aren't allowed to eat beets?' I'm not sure if this is a food myth or a request! Most of my clients seem to think beets (and carrots) are very high in sugar and will cause their blood sugars to spike. I ask the first of a series of questions: Do you normally eat beets? Do you even like beets? Do you find yourself overeating beets when you do eat them? Do you cook beets in a way that would add many unexpected carbohydrates to the meal (such as cooked with maple syrup and served with marshmallows)? When a client says, 'Yes, I like beets.' I try to pause and review the facts of the situation. One cup of cooked beets has about 15 grams of carbohydrates and 3 grams of fiber. Beets are therefore a food that is a good source of fiber. The greens are richer in iron, calcium, and vitamins A and C. Beetroots are an excellent source of folic acid and a very good source of manganese, potassium, and fiber. Both the greens and roots are a good source of phosphorus, magnesium, iron, and vitamin B.

"However, I often add, 'Don't trust ME!' Learn for yourself: create an experiment. Test your blood sugar before eating beets and then check two hours after. If your blood sugar is in the target range (typically less than 160 mg/dl), then that amount of beets, eaten with the other foods in your meal, is not an issue.

"The myth that this story is showing is the idea that there are foods you can and can't eat. All foods can be included as part of a healthy diet. There are no 'perfect' foods or 'evil' foods. You should avoid foods you dislike. You should eat foods that you enjoy eating. The enjoyment of food is a complex equation and it is greater than the immediate taste of the food. Ideally food selection considers both your personal preferences and situations surrounding socialization of the meal (who you are eating with) and your immediate and long-term health goals."

Myth #9   People with Diabetes Can't Drink Alcohol

The same guidelines for alcohol that apply to the general public also apply to most people with diabetes: If you want to drink alcohol, do so in moderation. However, if you take medications and have other medical issues that might interact negatively with alcohol, check with your health care provider as a precaution.

Moderation is defined by the U.S. Government's Dietary Guidelines for Americans and other organizations as no more than two drinks a day for men and one drink a day for women. One drink is defined as: 12 ounces of beer, 5 ounces of wine, 1.5 ounces of hard liquor (distilled spirits).

Alcohol has 7 calories per gram. Some alcoholic beverages, including wine, contain a small amount of carbohydrate. All types of alcohol have been shown to have some heart-health benefits: raising HDL (good) cholesterol and improving insulin resistance.

The biggest concern about alcohol intake is low blood sugar several hours after drinking if you take one or more blood glucose-lowering medications that can cause low blood sugar. If you don't take a blood glucose-lowering medication that can cause low blood sugar, then hypoglycemia should not be a concern. To prevent hypoglycemia when you drink alcohol, consume some food along with it, because alcohol lowers blood glucose levels less if you eat at the same time.

Myth #10   People with Diabetes Can't Eat Potatoes, Rice, Bread, and Pasta

People with diabetes don't have to give up potatoes; just make them a part of a balanced meal. When potatoes (or any starchy vegetable) are part of a meal, try to balance the plate by including nonstarchy vegetables such as a lettuce salad, green beans, or broccoli.

Potatoes are rich in nutrients. For example, they're higher in potassium than bananas, and they also provide dietary fiber and are good sources of vitamin C. When eating potatoes, remember portion size and be honest about quantity. One serving of potatoes is roughly the size of your fist, or about 1/2 cup. Baked and boiled potatoes are the healthiest choices. Instead of opting for potato chips or mashed potatoes loaded with butter and sour cream, try salsa, spicy mustard, or Greek yogurt to boost flavor.

To make oven-fried potatoes: Cut 4 medium potatoes or sweet potatoes lengthwise into wedges. Drizzle the wedges with one tablespoon olive oil or canola oil. Bake wedges in an even layer on a baking sheet at 375° F for 50 minutes. Makes 4 servings. *Per serving*: 164 calories, 3.5 grams total fat (0 grams saturated fat), 0 milligram cholesterol, 8 milligram sodium, 31 grams carb (1 gram sugars, 2 grams fiber), 4 grams protein.

Instead of potatoes, sweet potatoes are a great choice for people with diabetes and are in fact considered a "Diabetes Superfood."

DIABETES SUPERFOODS

The American Diabetes Association recommends including these superfoods in your meal plan:

- **Beans:** Whether you prefer kidney, pinto, navy, or black beans, you can't find more nutritious foods than beans. Their high fiber content gives you nearly one-third of your daily requirement in just 1/2 cup. Beans also are good sources of magnesium and potassium, important nutrients for people with diabetes. Although they are considered starchy vegetables, a 1/2 cup provides as much protein as an ounce of meat without the saturated fat. Use canned varieties to save time, but rinse first to remove excess sodium.
- **Dark green leafy vegetables:** These powerhouse foods such as spinach, collards, and kale are so low in calories and carbohydrates, you can eat as much as you want.
- **Citrus fruit:** Grapefruit, oranges, lemons, and limes provide part of your daily dose of soluble fiber, important for heart health, and vitamin C.
- **Sweet potatoes:** This starchy vegetable is packed full of fiber and vitamin A (as carotenoids), important for vision health. Try these in place of regular potatoes *for a lower glycemic index alternative.*
- **Berries:** Blueberries, strawberries, and other varieties are packed with antioxidants, vitamins, and fiber. Make a parfait alternating the fruit with light, nonfat yogurt for a new favorite dessert.
- **Tomatoes:** Everyone can find a favorite with this old standby. No matter how you like your tomatoes (pureed, raw, or in a sauce), you're eating vital nutrients like vitamin C, iron, and vitamin E.

(continued)

DIABETES SUPERFOODS (continued)

- **Fish with omega-3s:** Salmon, albacore tuna, mackerel, halibut, and herring are high in omega-3 fatty acids, which are important for heart health. Stay away from the breaded and deep-fried fish. They don't count toward your goal of 6 to 9 ounces of fish per week.
- **Whole grains:** These grains, such as pearled barley and oatmeal, are loaded with fiber, potassium, magnesium, chromium, omega-3 fatty acids, and folate. The germ and bran of the whole grain contain the important nutrients a grain product has to offer. Processed grains, like bread made from enriched wheat flour, do not have these vital nutrients.
- **Nuts:** An ounce of nuts can go a long way in providing key healthy fats along with hunger management. Nuts also give you a dose of magnesium and fiber. Some nuts and seeds, such as walnuts and flax seeds, also contain omega-3 fatty acids.
- **Fat-free milk and yogurt:** Everyone knows dairy can help build strong bones and teeth. In addition to calcium, many fortified dairy products are a good source of vitamin D. More research is emerging on the connection between vitamin D and good health. Pick the low-fat milk and low-fat yogurt as they have fewer carbs and are preferable for diabetics.

Myth #11   People with Diabetes Should Not Eat Fruit

While it's true that any food that contains carbohydrate (including fruit) will raise blood sugar, it doesn't mean you should eliminate healthy sources of carbohydrate from your diet. One way to help keep your blood glucose under control is to make sure your portions of carbohydrate-containing foods aren't too large. When choosing fruit, opt for fresh fruit, frozen fruit with no added sugar, or canned fruit in light syrup or 100 percent fruit juice.

The Dietary Guidelines for Americans recommends that everyone, including people with diabetes, eat about two cups of fruit per day. Fruits and vegetables, whether fresh, frozen, or canned, are excellent sources of much-needed vitamins, minerals, and dietary fiber. In fact, most people don't eat enough fruits and vegetables, which provide essential nutrients such as vitamins A and C, potassium, and magnesium. Fruits and vegetables are also relatively low in calories.

- One serving of *fruit* (one small piece or half of a large piece) has 15 grams of carbs and 60 calories.
- One serving of *nonstarchy vegetables* (1/2 cup cooked) has 5 grams of carbs and 25 calories.
- One serving of *starchy vegetables* (1/2 cup cooked) contains 15 grams of carbs and 80 calories.

Riva Greenberg says, "People tell me all the time they eat fruit because that's healthy but they don't realize many fruits are high in carbohydrates and will raise blood sugar. A friend told me her neighbor who has type 2 diabetes sits down with a huge bowl of fruit on his lap every night after dinner and couldn't understand why his blood sugar would skyrocket over 300 mg/dl. So as much as I like fruit, and as healthy as it is, I limit myself from overindulging.

"I most enjoy summer fruit and that's when I eat most of it—berries of all kinds, strawberries, raspberries, blueberries. Luckily they happen to not contain as much carbohydrate even though they taste so sweet, and they're packed with antioxidants. I get my blast of fruit in my morning oatmeal every day. I add a bit of green apple, blueberries, and maybe a bite of peach, plums, or figs—whatever's in the house. Then I take my morning walk around my local park. It takes an hour and by the time I'm home I often need a little more sugar to raise my blood sugar. That's my time to indulge in a few more bites of that peach or plum."

Rachel Garlinghouse believes in a total food revolution, "When I was diagnosed, I was told by medical professionals (and I read in various diabetes publications) that a diabetic can eat all the foods that a nondiabetic can, as long as I take enough insulin to cover what I'm consuming. But the diabetic's system, particularly a person with type 1 like myself, is complicated. 'Just take enough insulin' isn't the only factor in balancing one's blood sugar, nor is it practical advice. And the truth is that what the general population is consuming might very well lead them to a diabetes diagnosis. What needs to happen is a complete food revolution for everyone, not just a diabetic. Medical professionals need to stop sugar-coating (no pun intended) the seriousness of poor diet—for the diabetic and nondiabetic. Sadly, many medical professionals have very little nutritional education. Doctors take multiple classes on pharmaceuticals, but sometimes only one class on nutrition. How backward is that?"

Q&A WITH AMY CAMPBELL

Someone who does know a lot about eating right for diabetics is Amy Campbell, MS, RD, LDN, CDE, nutritionist at Joslin Diabetes Center and co-author of *16 Myths of a "Diabetic Diet."*

Amy, Please tell me about your motivation to write a book about the myths of a diabetic diet. Why are there still so many myths and what can we do to help educate people about eating right with diabetes?

After working for many years with patients who had type 1 and type 2 diabetes, my colleague Karen Chalmers and I were amazed by the prevalence of myths surrounding what people with diabetes can eat.There just wasn't much information out there and we wanted to clear up the misconceptions.The American Diabetes Association asked us to write a book about these common myths in 1999, and we completed a revised version in 2007.

Why do you think these myths are so hard to dispel?

I think a lot of people still don't see a CDE or a dietitian and may only see their primary care doctor for their diabetes management. I think a lot of people were taught one thing years ago, and habits are hard to change. There are also a lot of "experts" out there who are promoting myths about eating right with diabetes. People like celebrity fitness trainers or even Dr. Oz, who is very popular because he's on TV, sometimes perpetuate these myths.

Talk to me about the whole low-carb controversy in the diabetes world. If we have insulin to cover what we eat, why should we limit carbs? One of the myths that seems to surround carb intake and diabetes is that too much insulin is a bad thing. Can you help clarify or explain the differences of opinion?

New research continues to refute older findings and that can be hard for people with diabetes to keep up with. Many people with type 1 have found success with lower carb diets and are passionate and adamant about this type of eating because it has worked for them. However, while low carb might be right for some people, there are also people who do well with a vegetarian or a vegan diet, which tends to be higher in carbs. It's really about what works for you and what you can stick with over the years. Eating eggs for breakfast every day of the week is not for everyone.

I feel like there is confusion about the best way to eat for people with diabetes because the group of people under the umbrella term "diabetes" is so large. Can we talk about eating right for people with type 1 and type 2, or do we need to treat them differently? Do people with type 1 and type 2 diabetes share the same challenges and therefore similar solutions, or is one about weight loss and the other matching carbs to insulin?

When people are first diagnosed it can be very overwhelming, and the first thing we do is teach the basics of survival skills to eating right for both type 1 and type 2 diabetes. We teach patients how to make healthy food choices, then how to count carbohydrates and then we look at labels and carb guidelines. Once patients are ready to learn more we get specific and examine different goals for people with type 1 and type 2 diabetes. Goals for type 2 are more often to lose weight and look at portion control while type 1 may need to learn how to determine their insulin-to-carb ratios. At this point, when the patient is ready, it becomes about fine-tuning and the eating plan is individualized.

How beneficial or necessary are sugar-free and diabetes food products (Glucerna, Boost, Extend, etc.)?

I would say that it depends on the product. Sometimes these "diabetic foods" can be helpful and we've used Boost products in a weight loss program at Joslin with success, but in general, I would say they aren't usually necessary and for some people, they can be expensive. Also, many people won't use them correctly and will drink a shake with their meal (instead of as their meal), which defeats the whole purpose.

What is the biggest barrier to eating right for people with diabetes?

I think it's hard to make the change from your former lifestyle. I think always having to think about counting carbs wears on people and that's a big barrier to eating right. There are so many different messages about nutrition in general (don't eat carbs, yes eat carbs). People want to be told what to eat and there is no right answer. I think its important to take a break every now and then from logging your food intake and/ or blood sugars to avoid this frustration. If you see your blood sugars go up, take a walk, it's not the end of the world. Especially when it comes to the holidays, people get stressed out thinking about what they can and can't eat and it helps to realize that Thanksgiving and Christmas are just a few days out of the year. If your blood sugar is high one day, you can get back on track the next day.

Can you tell me how people with diabetes can benefit from the updated USDA MyPlate?

I think it's important to remember that eating right is not just about carbohydrates. We need to focus on eating a variety of healthy foods and sometimes we get so focused on the carbs that we forget everything else.

After twenty-six years of living with type 1 diabetes, I've finally come to realize that a "diabetic diet" is a great meal plan for everyone, whether they make their own insulin or not. Throughout my life I've run into people who, when they learn I have diabetes, will say, "But how can that be, you look so healthy?" I've stopped rolling my eyes in response and now use these conversations as opportunities to educate the public about diabetes, the differences between type 1 and type 2 diabetes, and the similarities, that we all have to eat well, exercise, and take our medication to live well with diabetes. I look healthy because I have diabetes. If it wasn't for diabetes, I don't know if I would eat as well as I do or exercise every day. I do those things out of habit, because they make me feel good and because I have diabetes. I tell people that the "diabetic diet," one of moderation, is the healthiest around.

AUTHENTIC ADVICE ON MANAGING MYTH

■ *My cousin taught me a saying that has proven to be helpful and easy to digest (pun!) for people. "I'm picky, but not by choice."* ■ Alyssa Rosenzweig

(continued)

AUTHENTIC ADVICE ON MANAGING MYTH (continued)

■ I just like to educate people and let them know that basically I have been trained in all things pancreas and I act as my own personal organ. With insulin and proper food choices I can make the necessary changes externally like their bodies do automatically internally. This way I am able to enjoy mint Oreo truffles and turtle cheesecake like every mother needs every now and then! Although, often I think most people roll their eyes and don't believe me because their great aunt twice removed had diabetes and couldn't eat any sugar at all or she would die. ■ Melissa Coffey

2   Diagnosed with Diabetes Means Becoming Your Own Nutritionist

When it comes to food, I'm constantly learning and evolving. For example, until yesterday, I had no idea that onions were high in carbohydrates. I use onions all the time in my cooking and have never accounted for them in my carb estimation. I have never been a very good carb counter; ever since I was first diagnosed, my eyes used to blur and my brain would start to zone out at the whole idea of counting carbs. When I went to my endocrinologist appointments they would ask me whether I used a "sliding scale" and what my carb-to-insulin ratio was, and I always shrugged. "I don't know," I'd say. "I just eat the same thing every day and give the same shot." Looking back now I realize my approach to eating was both restrictive and boring. Who wants to eat the same thing day after day? My A1Cs were okay, so none of my doctors got too fired up about my seemingly lackadaisical approach to carb counting. I figured my blood sugar swings were just part of living with diabetes. It was a grin-and-bear-it kind of attitude, because I didn't want to count my food intake. I didn't want to spend time thinking about what I was eating. Food was no longer a source of pleasure for me—it was a means to an end. And while diabetes made me feel like I had no control over my body, refusing to count carbs like a scientist gave me back some form of control.

I'm older and wiser now, and have a much better appreciation for and understanding of how food works. I eat well, and I eat in moderation, and I exercise almost every day. But I'm also still learning and am frequently reminded of how little I know about food. Learning that onions were a high carb vegetable was one of the recent epiphanies. I also used to think that I ate a diet relatively low in carbohydrates until I interviewed Riva Greenberg for a story in *Diabetes Health* magazine. Riva explained that she, too, used to think that she ate low-carb meals, but then realized her diet consisted of high carb, low glycemic index foods. She talked about how she sometimes indulged in pretzels (not the giant, hot pretzels you get at baseball games, but the regular kind you find at the grocery store), and I thought, really, pretzels are your indulgence? I always buy Snyders pretzels at the store and dip them in hummus or cream cheese for a snack. But my conversation with Riva got me thinking that maybe I wasn't as low carb as I thought.

I remember another conversation several years ago with my aunt, who was an avid runner and conscientious about her weight and suggested that if I ate fewer carbs, maybe I wouldn't need as much insulin. This was at the beginning of the whole low-carb craze and the Atkins diet and all she was eating was burgers with no buns. Who wanted a burger without a bun? I told her she was crazy.

"I have to eat carbs," I said. "If I don't, I'll get low!" I remember feeling very defensive and thinking, of course I have to eat carbs, I'd always eaten carbs, I'd always been told to eat carbs by my doctors and nutritionists, right? Right? I shrugged off my aunt's words; she didn't have diabetes and therefore didn't know what she was talking about. But her words lingered in the back of my mind.

Ever since I was diagnosed with type 1 diabetes in 1985, I was taught that the best diet for a diabetic was one of moderation. The recommended Standard American Diet suggested that 60 percent to 70 percent of caloric intake come from carbohydrates. On a side note, isn't it interesting, by the way, that the abbreviation for the Standard American Diet is SAD? As someone who loves language and talked about the language of illness in *The Smart Women's Guide to Diabetes*, I think "SAD" says a lot about this way of eating. Today some updates have been made and one of those updates includes the USDA's MyPlate guide.

Lesley Hoffman Goldenberg was diagnosed in 1994, and says she also remembers learning the exchange system for "things were classified as breads and proteins. I think a slice of bread was 15 grams of carbs so I learned to count things in 15 gram increments. I have always had a pretty strict 'don't eat' list of things I've tried over the years that have totally and completely messed up my blood sugar for hours. These items include: donuts, smoothies, muffins (the delicious, fluffy looking kinds at those awesome bakeries), frozen drinks, pancakes, etc. I also rarely eat full fat regular yogurt or gelato. I remember every week between junior high and Hebrew school, my mom would take me and my friends to Dairy Queen to get a snack before going to the synagogue. After I was diagnosed with diabetes, my mom felt strongly that we shouldn't change our routine of going to DQ with friends before Hebrew school. So, I changed my order slightly to a fudge bar (calories and carbs were written on the box) and we asked them if I could have one slice of cheese for my protein. The employees at DQ were happy to help us so my regular order at DQ became an ice cream bar and a slice of cheese!"

Sysy Morales, founder of The Girl's Guide to Diabetes website, was also diagnosed in 1994 at the age of 11. "I was told not to have any sugar, but I was encouraged to eat plenty of complex carbohydrates. I met with a diabetes educator and dietitian and both told me that I could have pancakes for breakfast but no syrup, I could have pasta, pizza, mashed potatoes but never dessert. I was encouraged to use a lot of artificial sweeteners and to drink diet soda. This worked out okay for blood sugar management because I used regular and NPH insulin and followed a strict schedule of meals and snacks, consistent carbohydrate load in meals and snacks, and scheduled insulin shots. As far as freedom and flexibility go, this really was difficult for me as a child. I went to birthday parties and often couldn't have anything to eat. After my soccer games, I didn't get to eat orange slices or have a juice box. On Halloween, I trick-or-treated and then my parents bought my bag of candy and my dad took it to work to give to coworkers."

Michelle Sorensen was diagnosed with type 1 diabetes in 1999. "I was educated about the Canadian Food Plan, with its different exchanges and food groups. I was instructed to cut out sugar in my tea and use artificial sweetener. Something I would never touch now!"

When I asked her why she would never touch artificial sweeteners, I didn't really want to know what she was going to say because I loved my daily coffee and Sweet and Low habit. She explained, "I just think those artificial sweeteners are trouble for so many reasons. A university friend of mine who majored in chemistry said no chemist would ever use them … they are so toxic. I was a big tea drinker, and from a diabetic perspective, I think it would have made more sense to just account for a teaspoon of sugar every morning in my insulin dose. What I noticed is that they [artifical sweeteners] make everything SO sweet that if anything, it probably messes with your perception of how sweet things should be. In terms of digestion, I believe they may have contributed to the digestive issues that developed in my first year with diabetes, but of course I could never know for sure. Nowadays I am very suspicious of anything that is not natural, but back then I kind of followed the advice of medical professionals and trusted they were right."

Michelle was taught to count carbohydrates and include a dairy, a protein, a carbohydrate, and fruit or vegetable with each meal. "At the time I ate a pretty healthy diet based on the Standard American Diet. I increased my dairy and ate a lot of crackers and cheese after having a sugar low, because I was told these were good foods for regulating my sugars. I ended up gaining some weight, although I was underweight when diagnosed. Before long, I started having digestive issues, which I now believe were partly caused by the changes I made. I was mixing foods and focusing more on counting carbs than on how hungry I was."

Riva Greenberg was diagnosed in 1972, and remembers being told she could no longer eat desserts. "Somehow the thought that I'd never have a candy bar again taunted me. Yet, of course, almost four decades ago, no one thought starchy foods raised blood sugar as much as sweet foods. So, since I was diagnosed my freshman year of college and I was living away from home—you guessed it—pizza was regularly on the dinner menu and foot-long tuna subs were a study night tradition! Of course since there were also no meters, I had no idea my beloved subs were raising my blood sugar off the charts."

When Aliza Chana Zaleon was diagnosed in 2001, she was told to eat three meals a day and three snacks a day. "I was on MDI [multiple daily injections], and I remember having to be strict about making sure that I actually *ate* a meal, and did so within the right amount of time after taking my insulin (I was on Humalog/NPH, then tried the 'easy' way of 70/30 premix which never quite worked, Lantus gave awesome control, but an allergic reaction even while in the PedICU on lots of IV prednisone, Novolog, and Regular. So I settled for Humalog/NPH mix until I started pumping). I was told to count carbs and limit them to two servings per meal, snacks should have one carb serving and one or two protein servings. I was in a medical center where they were transitioning over to thinking that you match the insulin to the meal, not the meal to the insulin, for which I was incredibly thankful! I was on a lot of different medications that made me crave sweets and other carb-heavy foods, and my endocrinologist was amazing about getting me through those times. Her attitude was that we just would adjust my insulin accordingly while I was on prednisone. I was lucky in that no medical professional ever told me any food was off limits."

Carbohydrate counting has replaced the food exchange list, and the USDA's updated *MyPlate* recommends:

Balancing Calories:
- Enjoy your food, but eat less.
- Avoid oversized portions.

Foods to Increase:
- Make half your plate fruits and vegetables.
- Make at least half your grains whole grains.
- Switch to fat-free or low-fat (1 percent) milk.

(continued)

MyPlate Recommendations (*continued*)
Foods to Reduce
■ Compare sodium in foods like soup, bread, and frozen meals—and choose the foods with lower numbers.
■ Drink water instead of sugary drinks.

Riva Greenberg says, "MyPlate is now the quintessential guide for healthy eating: a plate divided into quarters of slightly varying sizes representing how to create a healthy meal. It contains a larger quarter for vegetables, slightly smaller for grains, and slightly smaller for both fruits and protein. The hope is that it will help eaters avoid oversized portions and eat more nutritious meals."

Secretary of Agriculture Tom Vilsack reported, in a 2011 press release announcing the launch of the MyPlate icon, that after almost twenty years of preaching nutrition through a food pyramid that U.S. Department of Agriculture officials now say was overly complex, obesity rates have skyrocketed. "The new symbol is simple and gives diners an idea of what should be on their plates when they sit down at the dinner table. In fact, it appears only one-quarter of people who recognize the food pyramid ever used it. Further surveys show people are confused about what they should eat and most have no concept of portion sizes or balancing calories for weight control."

Nutritionist Amy Campbell says the MyPlate method is easy. "The 2005 food pyramid was a little complicated. All those vertical stripes in different colors. What did they mean? Sure, they were a guide to help consumers figure out how much of a particular food group to eat, but that somehow backfired. At least the original food pyramid was divided up into layers, but again, it left more than a few people scratching their heads as to what those layers really meant." In Campbell's opinion the plate is also balanced. "Take a look at the new plate if you haven't done so already. Note that it's divided into four sections: vegetables, fruits, grains, and protein. On the side is dairy. No longer are fat and sugar represented. Now, you may or may not agree with the proportions of the plate, and some of you may not drink milk or eat meat, for example, but it's hard to refute that the food groups aren't represented. In fact, the sections of the plate aren't necessarily supposed to be proportional because everyone is different in terms of what their nutritional needs are. Keep in mind that the plate is a general guideline to help get you started."

In her *Diabetes Self-Management* blog, Amy offers the following tips for using the MyPlate Guide:

- *Use a 9-inch plate if you're interested in controlling your weight and your blood glucose. Many plates these days are about 12 inches in diameter, which means you're likely to fill your plate with more food, which means more calories consumed, which means weight gain, which means ... you get the point.*

- *Yes, fruits, grains, and milk (or yogurt) are carbohydrates, and when you have diabetes, portions of these foods need to be controlled. But you don't have to cut them out. Fresh fruit, a lot of vegetables, and whole grains such as brown rice, quinoa, and whole wheat bread can definitely be part of a diabetes eating plan. Also, if you think milk or yogurt is too high in carbohydrate, try Greek-style yogurt, which contains more protein and less carbohydrate than regular yogurt.*

- *The new Dietary Guidelines advise people to consume no more than 2,300 milligrams of sodium per day, but if you are fifty-one years old or older, are African American, and/or have high blood pressure, diabetes, or kidney disease, your goal is no more than 1500 milligrams of sodium per day. Keeping your sodium intake that low is no small feat, but it can be done. It will mean becoming an expert label reader and choosing more fresh, fewer processed foods. As far as those sugary drinks go, shy away from them and go for water, seltzer water, or tea.*

MyPlate is similar to the American Diabetes Association's "Create Your Plate." Counting carbohydrates is a necessary evil of diabetes management. Whether you eat a greater or lesser amount of carbs, you've still got to know approximately how many are in what you eat in order to balance the carbs with the correct amount of insulin.

- Create Your Plate is a fast and easy way to choose and eat the foods you want.
- First focus on your portion sizes. Then make healthier food choices.
- Six simple steps to get started.
- Apply a similar method at breakfast.

Amy Campbell says, "Often, when people are diagnosed with diabetes, they don't know where to begin. One way is to change the amount of food you are already eating. Focus on filling your plate with nonstarchy vegetables and having smaller portions of starchy foods and meats. Creating your plate is an easy way to get started with managing blood glucose levels."

MyPlate doesn't work for everyone. Sysy Morales says, "I definitely do not follow the MyPlate recommendations. First of all, I think that those recommendations are very general and probably for the typical male. Being a petite female, I'm aware I don't need as many carbs or calories as they recommend. If I do what they recommend, and I have in the past, I become overweight. My typical breakfast is an egg and one piece of whole grain toast. Lunch is usually a salad with some chicken or tuna, olive oil, and vinegar. Dinner is often a little brown rice and green vegetables. My desserts and snacks are mostly fruit and dark chocolate."

The ADA offers six steps to *Create Your Plate.*

SIX EASY STEPS

Create Your Plate is simple and effective for both managing diabetes and losing weight. Creating your plate lets you still choose the foods you want, but changes the portion sizes so you are getting larger portions of nonstarchy vegetables and a smaller portion of starchy foods. When you are ready, you can try new foods within each food category.

Using your dinner plate, put a line down the middle of the plate.

1. On one side, cut it again so you will have 3 sections on your plate.
2. Fill the largest section with nonstarchy vegetables such as: spinach, carrots, lettuce, greens, cabbage, bok choy, green beans, broccoli, cauliflower, tomatoes, salsa, onion, cucumber, beets, okra, mushrooms, peppers, and turnip.
3. Now in one of the small sections, put starchy foods such as: whole grain breads, such as whole wheat or rye; whole grain, high-fiber cereal; cooked cereal such as oatmeal, grits, hominy, or cream of wheat; rice; pasta; dal; tortillas; cooked beans and peas, such as pinto beans or black-eyed peas; potatoes; green peas; corn; lima beans; sweet potatoes; winter squash; low-fat crackers or snack chips, pretzels, or fat-free popcorn.
4. And then on the other small section, put your meat or meat substitutes such as: chicken or turkey without the skin; fish such as tuna, salmon, cod, or catfish; other seafood such as shrimp, clams, oysters, crab, or mussels; lean cuts of beef and pork such as sirloin or pork loin; tofu; eggs; low-fat cheese
5. Add an 8 oz. glass of nonfat or low-fat milk. If you don't drink milk, you can add another small serving of carb such as a 6 oz. container of light yogurt or a small roll.
6. Add a piece of fruit or a half-cup of fruit salad and you have your meal planned. Examples are fresh, frozen, or canned in juice; frozen in light syrup; or fresh fruit.

Aliza Chana Zaleon follows the ADA's Create Your Plate as much as she can. Although she is "not able to eat as much as the typical person." Here's her plan:

For breakfast: "1/3 cup breakfast potatoes. 1 egg white plus 1 teaspoon of the yolk. 2 tablespoons of chopped onions and 2 tablespoons of minced garlic all sauteed in a pan until cooked, then add in the egg white and partial yolk; scramble lightly, and then add ¼ shredded mozzarella (part skim) cheese. If I'm in a hungry mood, I will add one piece of garlic cheese Texas toast on the side."

For lunch: "I have tortilla chips with melted shredded Mexican blend cheese with light sour cream on the side."

For dinner: "I have a kosher chicken breast, pounded out flat and then cut into bite size chunks. Then the chunks are 'marinated' in a beaten egg with 2 tablespoons of corn starch added. I then dip the chunks in matzo meal and sauté them lightly in a pan with canola oil. When cooked, I take the chunks out of the pan and put them in an oven-safe pan and I pour General Tso's sauce that I've made over the chunks and bake the chicken. In the frying pan, I then sauté some onions and garlic and frozen peas and scramble an egg. I add the rice to the pan and then soy sauce and let the rice absorb some of the flavors from the pan, and I have fried rice. A homemade Chinese food dinner!"

COUNTING CARBS

I think one of the biggest challenges to eating right with diabetes is dispelling some of the confusing myths about food. Instead of feeling overwhelmed by the nutritional information available, I think it's important to take it slow when it comes to educating yourself about eating right. One of the biggest advantages in the last decade for people with diabetes is the Food and Drug Administration's insistence on nutrition labeling. When I was first diagnosed, nutrition labels were hard to find and if you wanted to figure out what you were eating, you had to pull out your little paperback book.

Today, all that has changed, and even McDonald's gives you the nutritional content of your double cheeseburger. There are a variety of great iPhone apps that can help you determine the carb count in your food. There are also websites like CalorieKing with nutritional information for a wide variety of foods.

There are many carbohydrate-counting apps available today with more coming into the market every day. Some of the most popular are:
- GoMeals
- Carb Counting with Lenny
- CarbsControl
- WaveSense Diabetes Manager
- Diabetes Log
- Carb Manager
- Low Carb Diet Assistant
- R-Kcal

But do your research online and find the best one for your needs.

Lesley Hoffman Goldenberg counts carbs, or she "tries her hardest to," for everything that she eats. "I often look things up on www.calorieking.com but I also spend a lot of time estimating how many carbs are in things I eat, especially when I'm in a restaurant. If I'm eating at home with my husband or a friend, I often measure things and am super classy while eating—for example, I'll measure 1/2 cup of refried beans and eat them right out of the cup! Otherwise I just wing it and hope for the best. It's one of the most challenging parts of diabetes, especially when foods are high in fat and the foods spike blood sugar later. I oftentimes wake up with high morning blood sugars because of a meal I ate the night before—it is endlessly frustrating."

Rachel Garlinghouse says she was taught to count carbs. "However, five years into my diagnosis, I rarely look up how many carbs are in, for example, an orange. I basically have it figured out—what I can and cannot eat based on how my body reacts to that particular food. I do not keep track of my carbs in terms of writing them down. I am very careful about what I eat and how much, which seems to be working well for me."

Aliza Chana Zaleon was taught to count carbs by both a nutritionist and a certified diabetes educator (CDE). "I had another class with both of them when I wanted to start the pump. I absolutely LOVE counting carbs, and I measure everything out at home to ensure that I have the correct number of carbs. Eating out is more difficult, and now that technology is so prevalent, I look up the nutritional information for my meals before I eat, and I have to estimate how much I have had to eat of the portions given."

Sysy Morales counts carbs and says she can't imagine what her diabetes management would be without it. "I learned during an hour with a dietitian who also spent time teaching my mom. I have always been really interested in health so it was a natural thing for me to really get into as a kid. I almost made it a challenging game to walk through the super market with my mom and try to guess the carb amount in random foods before checking the label to see if I was close. After a few years I became really good at it. Now that it's been seventeen years, I don't even think about it. I subconsciously carb count before I get ready to eat. I don't eat many complex carbs so I don't really have to count high amounts of carbs, anyway. If I didn't do it at all, I can't imagine how I'd manage my blood sugars. It's a really crucial element in my diabetes management."

Sysy Morales' younger sister Ana is twenty-one years old now, but was diagnosed when she was three years old and says she counts carbs almost without thinking at this point. "I learned how to count carbs at an early age when I attended Camp Too Sweet, a week-long summer day camp for children with diabetes. It was a good environment for learning how to count carbohydrates because we were always reminded to count before we ate and there were nurses around to help us at all times."

Riva Greenberg read Dr. Richard Bernstein's book *The Diabetes Solution* a dozen years ago and says, "I decided to vacuum a lot of carbs, particularly refined carbs, out of my diet. While I didn't reduce my carbs to the meager amount he suggests, I did get rid of scones, muffins, pretzels, chips, candy, cookies, and pies and my blood sugars stopped 'riding the rollercoaster.' That's not to say I don't have a bite of these now and then but basically I tossed them out of the house. Both my lunch and dinner are generally the same—half vegetables with some beans and protein. My breakfast is my only high carb meal, but again, complex carbs. Every time I mention it when I speak to patients everyone grabs a pen to write it down: steel cut oatmeal, flax seed, sunflower seeds, mix. Top with a bit of fruit, spoonful of peanut and almond butter, 0 percent fat plain Greek yogurt and low-fat cottage cheese. Chew, delight."

Michelle Sorensen says she is mindful of how many carbs she eats, and counts what she eats, "but not the same way I used to count them. In the early days I counted carbs, calculated my insulin dose and wrote it all down. Now I fill my plate with food and usually aim to include about 15 to 20 grams of low-GI [glycemic index] carbs, taking about 2 to 2.5 units of insulin for each meal. I am much more likely to have a high sugar from snacking and not taking enough insulin than I am from a meal."

MEETING WITH A NUTRITIONIST

Many people, when they are initially diagnosed with diabetes, meet with a certified diabetes educator, an endocrinologist and a nutritionist or dietitian. In the best cases, patients will continue to meet with this "diabetes team" for many years. However, many patients are seen only by their primary care doctor, who often does not have enough time to go over all the complex meal planning information. This is where a dietitian or nutritionist can be a great support.

When Lesley Hoffman Goldenberg was first diagnosed, she and her parents met with a diabetes team that included a diabetes educator, a social worker, and a nutritionist. "The nutritionist was initially helpful with identifying foods that were easy to count and easy on the blood sugar. As time went on, though, it was just easier for me to figure out carb counts with trial and error since no one nutritionist could help with all the foods I ate and all the places I visited. As an adult, I have met with a nutritionist, but again, it wasn't so helpful. I have become my own nutritionist, without the formal degree!"

Aliza Chana Zaleon believes that her post-diagnosis nutrition classes were really helpful. "We were taught to eat well-balanced meals with choices of protein, carbohydrate, vegetable, dairy (which often has a good bit of carb), where everything was measured out for correct serving size. We even had (and still to this day have) a digital food scale to weigh foods to get the correct serving of meats, cheese, poultry, and fish. Yes, my doctor sent me to a group diabetes nutrition class after diagnosis to learn about how food impacts blood glucose levels, and to talk about carb counting. I successfully completed that class, which was mainly to learn how to count carbohydrates accurately, I believe! I do follow the recommendations that I learned in that class each and every day. After the group class, I asked my doctor if I could see somebody one-on-one for nutrition goals, and she referred me to someone outside of the hospital system."

Michelle Sorensen met with a few dietitians in the early years. "I don't remember their recommendations clearly, but I do remember the focus on food groups and always feeling like I wasn't doing a great job of following the rules. I was very busy at that time of my life and really didn't make time for cooking. I would buy fruit and vegetables and they would often go bad before I ate them. I wish, in retrospect, that the kind of information they provided was more about holistic nutrition, helping me to think about increasing the value of my food rather than counting carbs."

Rachel Garlinghouse says she was "blessed" to meet with an outstanding dietitian who she still speaks with today, five years later. "She gave me a personalized meal plan and adjusted my plan based on my weight, food preferences, and activity levels. Over a year ago I became a vegetarian, so my dietitian helped me generate ways to get enough protein in my diet. When I was preparing to meet with the dietitian for the first time, I told myself if she wasn't someone who practiced what she preached (meaning she was clearly unhealthy), I was walking out. I wasn't going to take advice from yet another (I've seen plenty) bad medical professional. Luckily she was very fit and knowledgeable."

Ana Morales was so young when she was diagnosed that it was her parents that met with a nutritionist. "Several years later, however, I met with a nutritionist when I got an insulin pump. We first went over serving sizes and different ways to measure food and then moved on to the importance of eating foods from the different food groups, etc., etc. I don't even really remember what her recommendations for me were, probably because I was in eighth grade or so and at that point I wasn't having many problems with my diabetes control. I also didn't fully realize how important it was for me to control my diabetes. I didn't realize that part until much more recently, once things started to go downhill in terms of my control.

Once I started using the pump, I abused the freedom that came with it a bit. I snacked more because all I had to do was push some buttons and I was covered. I also entered high school within a year of using the pump (after being home schooled for three years) and the food I had for lunch wasn't always the healthiest. I ate things like pizza, corn dog nuggets, and peanut butter and jelly on white bread. I had a really hard time stomaching their salads that consisted of browning lettuce, so I rarely got them. Now I'm paying the price and re-learning which foods help keep me at the most stable blood sugar levels."

Ana is a college student and struggles to find foods that are healthy, affordable, and work well for blood sugar management. "I try to get foods that have easily visible ingredients such as salads and sandwiches. I always ask for cucumbers and wheat bread when I order my regular turkey sandwich and I've almost entirely eliminated creamy dressings from my salads. Now I just stick to oil, vinegar, and pepper. I eat vegetables but just a limited amount, so I'm trying to eat more. I've found that soups are a good way for me to eat vegetables so I have cans of vegetable soup in my closet at school. I'm really determined to make myself like broccoli because I've had this weird thing about wanting to eat it for the longest time ... I'm not sure why. Overall it's definitely been a process, but I just try to remember how crucial it is for me to keep myself as healthy as possible."

I asked Ana what she meant by "paying the price," and she explained that she has consistently had high A1Cs since high school, even getting up to a 10 once. "I've brought it down since then, but it still hasn't been as low as it should be. I gained about thirty pounds in high school, but I've lost about half of that since starting college (instead of the other way around). The last time I went to the dentist this past summer, I was warned about taking care of my gums because they weren't as healthy as they should be and I'm at risk for gum disease because of the diabetes." Ana uses her art as a form of therapy and contributes to the website A Girl's Guide to Diabetes, that she shares with her sister Sysy.

Diabetes Life has some great resources for eating right on their website, including slideshows that can be downloaded in a pdf version. In their "Best and Worst Foods for Blood Sugar" they say *Eat This, Not That*:

> EAT ... Scrambled eggs with vegetables and cheese. *Two scrambled eggs with a tablespoon of milk contains 197 calories and 1.5 grams of carbs. Add cheese and fresh, low-carb veggies to up the nutrient quota.*

> NOT ... An egg-white omelet on a "multi-grain" bagel. *For one thing, the vast majority of an egg's amazing array of nutrients are in the yolk, so keep it in there! Second, a multi-grain bagel is likely to have very little whole grain or fiber in it and a huge amount of carbs. Starbucks' Multigrain Bagel packs 62 grams, along with a whopping 320 calories.*

EAT … Greek yogurt or cottage cheese. *A 4-ounce serving of 4 percent milk fat cottage cheese has 6 grams of carbs (lower fat varieties will have more), 12 grams of protein, and 120 calories. Full-fat Greek yogurt contains about 4 grams of carbs per 4 ounces, 150 calories, and 8 grams of protein.*

NOT … Low-fat fruit yogurt. *Eight ounces of fat-free, fruit flavored yogurt contains 43 grams of carbs. Low-fat and fat-free yogurts are chockfull of hidden carbs and sugar; they need it to replace the fat! Stick to plain, full-fat yogurts or go for low-carb fruit versions.*

EAT … Whole fresh fruit. *A half-cup of fresh strawberries has 23 calories and 5.5 grams of carbs.*

NOT … A fruit smoothie. *A small Strawberry Fruit Coolatta from Dunkin' Donuts weighs in at 72 grams of carbs and 300 calories. Plus, fruit is best eaten the way it came from nature. The fibrous membranes, pulp, and flesh keep the sugars from being absorbed so quickly into your bloodstream.*

EAT … Crispbread. *One-half of a big slice of Wasa Whole Grain crispbread (5 grams of carbs) quenches a crunch craving without all the junk. Its ingredients are simply whole grain rye flour, water, yeast, and salt. For a snack, have a half topped with a soft cheese and some diced veggies.*

NOT … Rice cakes. *Confused? Aren't rice cakes a health food? Not really. One serving of salt and pepper mini rice cakes contains 11 grams of carbs and 70 calories. (To top if off, the fourth ingredient is "corn syrup solids," and the seventh ingredient is sugar! Is that really necessary?)*

EAT … Nuts. *One-quarter cup of nutrient-rich pistachios delivers 8.5 grams of carbs along with a healthy*

3 grams of fiber. Almonds are one of the lowest carb nut varieties; one-half cup of almonds contains just 3.6 grams of carbs.

NOT ... Snack mix. *One cup of cereal snack mix has 40 grams of carbs. There are a few nuts in the recipe, but most of this mix is made of refined flour and sugar (not to mention salt), in the form of cereal, pretzels, and bagel chips. Blood sugar disaster waiting to happen.*

EAT ... Barley. *Barley is the lowest glycemic grain tested so far, which means it has a more moderate effect on blood sugar than other grains. One-half cup of cooked, pearl barley contains 21.6 grams of carbs (3 grams of fiber) and 94 calories. And if you can find the less pro-cessed, hulled barley or Scotch barley, the carbs and gly-cemic index will be lower.*

NOT ... Rice. *Rice is a high-glycemic grain, unfortu-nately, and all varieties will cause blood sugar to rise fast. One-half cup of cooked white rice has 26.6 grams of carbs and no fiber to speak of. Go for barley or qui-noa. And if you choose rice, remember to go with brown rice, which is a nutritious whole grain.*

EAT ... Spaghetti squash. *A half cup of boiled or baked spaghetti squash has 19 calories and 4.7 grams of carbs. Here's a simple recipe: Spaghetti Squash with Herbs.*

NOT ... Pasta. *You may not need us to tell you this, but one cup of cooked spaghetti contains 43 grams of carbs. When it's pasta night, make sure you buy whole grain, low-carb noodles and keep portions small.*

EAT ... Dark chocolate mini chips. *One tablespoon of Hershey's semi-sweet miniature chocolate chips has 4 grams of carbs and 80 calories. Minis are the way to go; you'll be surprised how satisfying a small amount of these can be.*

NOT … Dried fruit. *A 1.5-ounce serving (one small box of raisins) of dried fruit has 34 grams of carbs. Stick to fruit in its fresh form.*

EAT … Popcorn. *One cup of air-popped popcorn has 6.2 grams of carbs and 31 calories. And popcorn is a whole, unprocessed food. Now that's a great snack.*

NOT … Potato chips. *One ounce (20 chips) of plain, thin potato chips contains 15 grams of carbs and 150 calories. Count out 20 chips, lay them next to about three cups of popcorn, and decide which is a better investment for your 15 grams of carbs.*

Meagan Esler was incorrectly diagnosed with type 2 diabetes when she was eighteen years old and says no matter how much she exercised and how little she ate, she still had high blood sugars. "When I was diagnosed with diabetes, I had never heard of a carbohydrate. I was told to limit them greatly since, at the time, they didn't know if I was type 1 or 2. I agreed, hoping to see gorgeous blood sugars appear on my glucose meter. Needless to say, I was disappointed. I ate less and less carbohydrates, and soon was subsisting on cheese, eggs, and salad. I was miserable! No matter how much I exercised and how limited my carbohydrates were, my blood sugars refused to stay in range. My weight was at an all time low and I was diagnosed with type 1 diabetes.

"I was relieved in a way with my diagnosis, because it meant I wasn't going crazy, that there was a reason that my sugars weren't cooperating. I needed insulin. I met with my diabetic educator and my nutritionist to learn to count carbohydrates and to come up with a meal plan that actually included them. I would be taking shots every day for the rest of my life, but on the upside, I'd be allowed to have a piece of cake on my birthday without having high blood sugar, and allowed to eat mashed potatoes on Thanksgiving without feeling totally left out.

"Today I eat about thirty carbohydrates per meal. I was eating sixty and up for years, but noticed my weight was going up a few pounds each year as I became more and more cozy with my beloved carbohydrates. I found that thirty carbs satisfy me, without overdoing it." Meagan's meal plan:

For breakfast: "I can have whole grain (Kashi) waffles or fruit with
   some low-fat cottage cheese or string cheese."
For lunch: "A whole grain sandwich."
For dinner: "Generally a salad with soup or a roll."

"I also incorporate a couple of low-carb snacks like nuts, low-fat cheese, or a variety of vegetables. My snacks are generally kept to 15 carbs or less. I'm slowly losing weight with reducing my carbohydrates and adding some exercise, and am pleased with the flexibility of my meals. Nothing is completely off limits, portions are just reduced."

Q&A WITH SUSAN WEINER

Susan Weiner RD, CDE, with a private practice in New York, is a contributing medical producer for *Diabetes Life* TV and serves as a member of *Diabetes Life*'s medical advisory board. She is the certified diabetes educator for diabetessisters.org, a nonprofit organization dedicated to the education and advocacy of women with diabetes. She is a valued contributor on a variety of nutrition topics—primarily weight management, diabetes, and polycystic ovary syndrome (PCOS). Further, Susan is a well-respected lecturer for organizations such as the American College of Sports Medicine, and was the official sports nutritionist for the American Diabetes Association's Walk America program. She was an adjunct professor of nutrition at Queens College for more than 13 years and taught at the Academy of Applied Personal Training Education at Hofstra University.

I remember when I was first diagnosed at fourteen years old, I was very overwhelmed and felt like I had to re-learn how to eat. How do you help patients overcome these feelings of anxiety about eating right?

When a person is first diagnosed with diabetes it can be overwhelming. Information is just "thrown" at a newly diagnosed person, and the person often shuts down. The first thing I do when meeting with people who are newly diagnosed is to "listen" to what they are typically eating, and what concerns they have about a diabetes eating plan. There is no-one-size-fits-all with eating for anyone, with or without diabetes. In order to lessen anxiety, we focus on what steps they can take to improve how they are feeling, and how to specifically control blood sugar through proper nutrition and physical activity. My patients have a say in what they eat. We discuss it, which reduces anxiety and gives them control over what they are eating. I'm not the diabetes food police. I just help a person with diabetes make better food choices. Until there is a cure for diabetes, managing what you eat, exercise, reducing stress and medications puts "you" in control. Control helps to reduce anxiety.

What is the first thing you teach a newly diagnosed person with diabetes? How to count carbs? The importance of weight loss? Understanding insulin-to-carb ratios?

Not everyone with diabetes needs to lose weight. While many people with prediabetes and diabetes are overweight, most people with type 1 have experienced a recent weight loss. Other people with prediabetes or type 2 might have attempted to lose weight (with some success) even before they start working with me. Depending on the individual situation (Is the person on insulin? Does that person need to lose weight? What kind of meds is the person taking?, Is he or she preparing meals or eating out? How are the person's blood sugars?) will help me determine where to begin with nutrition education.

There is a lot of controversy about eating carbohydrates. Can you describe your approach in regard to the American Diabetes Association's recommendation of 45 to 60 carbs per meal? Is this too much, or too little? Do we as patients pay too much attention to carbs in general?

Because people with diabetes either do not produce insulin, or might have insulin resistance, carbs have to be adjusted in most diets. People with diabetes should be following a healthy eating plan (as should people without diabetes). Therefore, I recommend blood sugar testing (fasting in the morning, and 2 hours post meals for people on insulin, or on an insulin-sensitizing medication). Check with your physician about how often to test blood sugar.

The amount of carbs that I recommend depends on a person's weight, blood sugars, medications, and exercise regime. If someone works out often (and at a high intensity), that person will require more carbohydrate than is recommended by the American Diabetes Association. However, if a person with diabetes is inactive, they will require less carbs during the day. I don't believe in a "one-size-fits-all" approach to meal management. I also recommend carbs that have nutritional value such as vegetables, fresh fruits, and whole grains. There is very little nutritional value in candy and cake, and I don't recommend that as part of an everyday meal plan (I consider those "sometimes" foods, which should only be eaten occasionally due to their poor nutritional content).

What is the biggest challenge to people with diabetes when it comes to eating right? And are there different challenges for type 1s and type 2s and pre-diabetics? How can we best get the message of eating right across to these varied groups?

I believe the biggest challenge to eating right is that diabetes never takes a day off. When a person without a medical condition wants to lose weight, they can "splurge" a bit on a holiday without serious blood sugar consequences. If you are on a medication for diabetes, or insulin, the timing of meals becomes very important. So a major challenge is how to manage your meds if your meal is delayed, or on a day when you are ill. Other times, lack of sleep can influence blood sugar levels. Once again, it is very important to check your blood sugar levels to make sure that you are managing your food correctly.

The challenges for type 1 and type 2 or pre-diabetics might be associated with taking insulin and weight control. Remember that many people with type 2 diabetes also take insulin to manage their diabetes. All people with diabetes have to be involved in their medical and nutritional management. So getting the word out in online communities or in local support groups is essential.

The American Diabetes Association's Create Your Plate is similar to the U.S. Department of Agriculture's MyPlate method. Can you describe how these visual aids are helpful for people with diabetes?

The plate method helps put meals in perspective. If you don't have the opportunity to weigh and measure specific portions, the plate method allows you to visually approximate serving sizes. I encourage my patients to weigh out serving sizes for a few weeks when they are diagnosed. After a while they can visually figure out a serving size, but the initial weighing and measuring gives them confidence when preparing meals. The plate method also encourages the consumption of vegetables, which are rich in vitamins, minerals, and fiber (and are low in calories).

What do you hope your patients take away from their time with you?

I hope my patients take the message that eating well for diabetes simply means eating well! Many of my patients comment that they are now eating better than they ever did before, because we focus on health and well-being. Until there is a cure for diabetes, proper nutrition, exercise, and stress management (along with insulin or meds as needed) are a joint effort between the patient and his or her health care team.

Turns out that my aunt Sue was onto something as far as carbo-hydrates go. I've begun to experiment with my diet and have found that the less carbs I eat, the less insulin I need, and if I'm careful, I don't have to worry (too much) about low blood sugars. Now, looking back at the advice I received from the medical community over the years, I get irritated. Why was I advised to include carbs as a necessary element to my diet? Why did I cling to the idea that I needed carbs to keep the lows at bay when what I really needed to keep the lows at bay was less insulin? It's like Susan says—we all need to focus on health and well-being. Eating right for people with diabetes is a model the rest of the country should follow.

AUTHENTIC ADVICE

- *To this day, I believe my dietitian is the most important person on my medical team. I think diabetics must be their own educator. I see several medical professionals—a gynecologist, a general practitioner, a podiatrist, a dentist, an optometrist/ophthalmologist, an endocrinologist, a dermatologist, and a dietitian—and I take their thoughts and advice seriously. However, at the end of the day, it's my body and my life. I am in charge of my disease. Therefore, I always walk into appointments armed with questions and concerns. It's up to me to be healthy and strong.* ■ Rachel Garlinghouse
- *The best way to count carbs is by looking at nutrition information on all the foods you eat until you can remember them without looking. You should also remember serving sizes so that you can adjust the amount of carbs if you have more or less than the serving size of a certain food.* ■ Ana Morales

3

"Best Diets"

I've been on a "diet" for twenty-six years. I'm tall and for most of my life I've been slim, yet as a woman with diabetes, I've always had to watch what I eat. Today, as a forty-one-year-old mom, I know that a diabetes diet (for lack of a better term) is a healthy way to eat, but it felt restrictive for a long time. As a woman with diabetes, food is not just food. Whether it's a slice of apple, a piece of broccoli, or a spoonful of peanut butter, I have to think about every bite that I put into my mouth. How many carbs? How much do I need to bolus? Can I eat red meat, and should I avoid dairy products? There are so many questions and an ongoing debate when it comes to what we should eat as women with diabetes, and that's why it's tempting when someone can eliminate the guesswork and tell us what to do.

In its second year of diet rankings, the *US News & World Report* named the DASH diet (Dietary Approaches to Stop Hypertension) as the Best Overall:

> *To create the second annual rankings,* US News *editors and reporters spent months winnowing potential additions to our diet roster and then mining medical journals, government reports, and other resources to create in-depth profiles for the five that made the cut.*
>
> *A panel of 22 nationally recognized experts in diet, nutrition, obesity, food psychology, diabetes, and heart disease reviewed our profiles, added their own fact-finding, and rated each diet in seven categories: how easy it is to follow,*

its ability to produce short-term and long-term weight loss,
its nutritional completeness, its safety, and its potential for
preventing and managing diabetes and heart disease.

One of those experts was Amy Campbell, a registered dietitian and certified diabetes educator at Joslin Diabetes Center, who helps develop and implement all aspects of diabetes education programs. Campbell serves as an advisory board member of CalorieKing, American's leading provider of calorie-centric education tools for food awareness, and is a registered dietitian advisor for the Egg Nutrition Center. She says, "I was excited to participate in this ranking because, representing Joslin Diabetes Center, it gave me an opportunity to hopefully help show that:

- Eating with diabetes doesn't have to be vastly different than eating when you don't have diabetes. Sure, you need to control portions and carbohydrate intake, but people need to know that healthy eating is pretty much the same for everyone, diabetes or not.
- There isn't a magic bullet or diet for someone with diabetes. There are many options, and as with any person, an eating plan for a person with diabetes needs to be individualized. The DASH plan may work for one person, whereas a vegan plan or Weight Watchers works for others. That's the beauty of participating in a ranking like this: one size doesn't fit all."

Campbell says, "Hopefully people with diabetes who read this guide will pick up the common themes of variety, balanced nutrition, lower saturated fat and sodium, and more fiber. There's the potential for someone to still feel overwhelmed, as there are many options, but the intent is to share these rankings with a dietitian or other health care provider in making a collaborative decision on what plan would work best for that particular person."

She adds, "The other point that I wanted to add is that the top five diabetes diets are actually, in my opinion, eating plans and not diets. Dukan, Atkins, and Paleo I view as being truly 'diets' in that most people follow them to lose weight (think of Kate Middleton losing weight on Dukan for her wedding). They're okay to follow briefly, but I doubt most people can really stick with that way of eating long term. Dietitians are big on advising people to choose an eating plan that they can follow long term, not just for a few months, and the top five 'diets' are really ways of eating for the long haul."

In general, the top five best diets (or plans) for diabetes had the following in common:

- Heart healthy
- Promote a variety of foods (and no one food group was overly restricted)
- Help with weight loss
- More nutritionally balanced than many of the other diets
- Not overly expensive to follow
- Not overly tedious or time consuming to follow, either
- Most are backed by research, showing that they help move certain biomarkers, such as LDL cholesterol, blood pressure, A1C and/or weight

"The Paleo and Dukan diets can certainly promote weight loss and will also likely lower A1C levels. However, these diets don't have much research behind them in terms of long-term safety, cardiovascular benefits, and long-term diabetes control," says Campbell. "The Dukan diet, initially, falls short on carbohydrate and fiber and is overly high in sodium. The Paleo diet also falls short in terms of carbs and is higher in fat and protein than is generally recommended. The other issue with these two diets is that they can be difficult to follow long term. Anyone can follow either of these diets for a limited amount of time, but due to their restrictive nature, meal preparation and eating out can be challenging, which, for many Americans, just isn't practical."

US News & World Report: Top Five Best Diabetes Diets 2012

1 Biggest Loser Diet
2 DASH Diet
3 Mayo Clinic Diet
4 Ornish Diet
5 Vegan Diet*

———

*Read more about the vegan/vegetarian Diet in Chapter 5.

The Paleo Diet Came in at #25 for Diabetes Diets

Most of the other diets are better options for preventing or controlling diabetes, according to experts' scores in this category. A lack of research showing its worth gave experts little option than to hand out poor scores, shooting it to the bottom of the bunch.

However, there has been a great deal of recent research that suggests a Paleo diet is good for people with diabetes. A study from Lund University in Sweden found markedly improved capacity to handle carbohydrate after eating such foods for three months.

What Is the Paleo Diet?

The Paleo or "Caveman" or "Stone Age" diet is based on the ancient diet from the Paleolithic era. Following this diet means cutting out refined sugar, dairy, legumes, and grains, and eating mainly meat, fish, poultry, fruits, and veggies.

Dr. Steve Parker, author of *Conquer Diabetes and Prediabetes: The Low-Carb Mediterranean Diet,* and *The Advanced Mediterranean Diet: Lose Weight, Feel Better, Live Longer,* says he started getting interested in the Paleo diet in 2011 when patients began asking questions. "This is a grassroots movement," he says.

"We are really in the infancy stage of understanding the Paleo diet."

A board-certified internist, Dr. Parker is interested in both the carbohydrate-restricted diet and the Mediterranean diet, and though he does not have diabetes himself, he has written extensively about the Paleo diet for people with diabetes. He says there is a huge variety of foods in the Paleo diet and that the biggest challenge for patients switching from the Standard American Diet (SAD) will be a reduction in carbs. Dr. Parker says 25 percent of the calories will be coming from protein and the fat content of the protein will vary depending on which version of the Paleo diet they are following. He has been unable to find evidence that shows a correlation between heart disease and fat consumption. He writes:

- *Some studies show no association between dietary saturated fats and coronary heart disease.*
- *Some studies associate lower rates of coronary heart disease with higher saturated fat intake.*
- *Higher saturated fat intake was associated with less progression of coronary atherosclerosis in women.*
- *Lowering saturated fat intake did not reduce total or coronary heart disease mortality.*

The scientific community is slowly moving away from the original Diet-Heart/Lipid Hypothesis. It is being replaced with stronger anti-atherosclerosis theories that promote:

- *Fruit and vegetable intake*
- *Whole grain intake*
- *Low glycemic index eating*
- *Increased consumption of plant oils and fish*
- *Moderate intake of nuts*
- *Moderate intake of low-fat dairy (e.g., DASH diet but there is less consensus on this point)*

*If you want to hedge your bets, go ahead and limit
your saturated fat intake. It probably won't hurt you.
It might help a wee bit. By the same token, I'm not
going on an all-meat and cheese, ultra-high-saturated
fat diet; I don't want to miss out on the healthy
effects of fruits, vegetables, whole grains, fish, nuts,
and low glycemic index carbohydrates. Some would
throw red wine into the mix. This "prudent diet"
reflects what I hereby christen "The 21st Century
Diet-Heart Hypothesis."*

*If you're worried about coronary heart disease and
atherosclerosis, spend less time counting saturated
fat grams and more time on other risk-reducing
factors: diet modification as above, get regular
exercise, control your blood pressure, achieve a
healthy weight, and don't smoke. More bang for the
buck.*

After our interview, Dr. Parker wrote a summary about the Paleo
diet for people with diabetes on his blog, *The Paleo Diabetic:*

*Fresh, minimally processed food. Meat (lean or not?
supermarket vs. yuppiefied?), poultry, eggs, fish, leafy
greens and other vegetables, nuts, berries, fruit, and
probably tubers.*

*Non-Paleo: Highly processed, grains, refined sugars,
industrial plant/seed oils, legumes, milk, cheese,
yogurt, salt, alcohol.*

Is the Paleo Diet Deficient in Any Nutrients?

*A quick scan of Loren Cordain's website found men-
tion of possible calcium and vitamin D deficits.
Paleoistas will get vitamin D via sun exposure and
fish (especially cold-water fatty fish). Obtain calcium*

from broccoli, kale, sardines, almonds, collards. (I wonder if the Recommended Dietary Allowance for calcium is set too high.)

What About Carbohydrates and Diabetes and the Paleo Diet?

Diabetes is a disorder of carbohydrate metabolism. In a way, it's an intolerance of carbohydrates. In type 1 diabetes, there's a total or near-total lack of insulin production on an autoimmune basis. In type 2 diabetes, the body's insulin just isn't working adequately; insulin production can be high, normal, or low. In both cases, ingested carbohydrates can't be processed in a normal healthy way, so they stack up in the bloodstream as high blood sugars. If not addressed adequately, high blood glucose levels sooner or later will poison body tissues. Sooner in type 1, later in type 2. (Yes, this is a gross over-simplification.)

Gluten-Rich Neolithic Food

If you're intolerant of lactose or gluten, you avoid those. If you're intolerant of carbohydrates, you could avoid eating them, or take drugs to help you overcome your intolerance. Type 1 diabetics must take insulin. Insulin's more optional for type 2s. We have eleven classes of drugs to treat type 2 diabetes; we don't know the potential adverse effects of most of these drugs. Already, three diabetes drugs have been taken off the U.S. market or severely restricted due to unacceptable toxicity: phenformin, troglitazone, and rosiglitazone.

Humans need two "essential" fatty acids and nine "essential" amino acids derived from proteins.

"Essential" means we can't be healthy and live long without them. Our bodies can't synthesize them. On the other hand, there are no essential carbohydrates. Our bodies can make all the carbohydrate (mainly glucose) we need.

Since there are no essential carbohydrates, and we know little about the long-term adverse side effects of many of the diabetes drugs, I favor carbohydrate restriction for people with carbohydrate intolerance. (To be clear, insulin is safe, indeed life-saving, for those with type 1 diabetes.)

That being said, let's think about the Standard American Diet (SAD) eaten by an adult. It provides an average of 2, 673 calories a day. Added sugars provide 459 of those calories, or 17 percent of the total. Grains provide 625 calories, or 23 percent of the total. And most of those sugars and grains are in processed, commercial foods. So added sugars and grains provide 40 percent of the total calories in the SAD.

Anyone going from the SAD to pure Paleo eating will be drastically reducing intake of added sugars and grains, our current major sources of carbohydrate. Question is, what will they replace those calories with?

That's why I gave a thumbnail sketch of the Paleo diet above. Take a gander and you'll see lots of low-carb and no-carb options, along with some carb options. For folks with carbohydrate intolerance, I'd favor lower-carb veggies and judicious amounts of fruits, berries, and higher-carb veggies and tubers. "Judicious" depends on the individual, considering factors such as degree of residual insulin production, insulin sensitivity, the need to lose excess weight, and desire to avoid diabetes drugs.

Compared to the standard "diabetic diet" (what's that?) and the Standard American Diet, switching to Paleo should lower the glycemic index and glycemic load of the diet. Theoretically, that should help with blood sugar control.

A well-designed low-carb paleo diet would likely have at least twice as much fiber as the typical American diet, which would also tend to limit high blood sugar excursions.

In general, I favor a carbohydrate-restricted Paleo diet for those with diabetes who have already decided to "go Paleo." I'm not endorsing any Paleo diet for anyone with diabetes at this point—I'm still doing my research. But if you're going to do it, I'd keep it lower-carb. It has a lot of potential.

Are There Any Immediate Dangers for a Person with Diabetes Switching to the Paleo Diet?

It depends on three things:

1. Current diet
2. Current drug therapy
3. The particular version of Paleo diet followed

Remember, the Standard American Diet provides 40 percent of total calories as added sugars and grains (nearly all highly refined). Switching from SAD to a low-carb Paleo diet will cut carb intake and glycemic load substantially, raising the risk of hypoglycemia if the person is taking certain drugs.

Who knows about carb content of the standard "diabetic diet"? Contrary to popular belief, there is no monolithic "diabetic diet." There is no ADA diet

(American Diabetes Association). My impression, however, is that the ADA favors relatively high carbohydrate consumption, perhaps 45 percent to 60 percent of total calories. Switching to low-carb Paleo could definitely cause hypoglycemia in those taking the aforementioned drugs.

One way to avoid diet-induced hypoglycemia is to reduce the diabetic drug dose.

A type 2 overweight diabetic eating a Standard American Diet—and I know there are many out there—would tend to see lower glucose levels by switching to probably any of the popular paleo diets. Be ready for hypoglycemia if you take those drugs.

Paleo diets are not necessarily low-carb. Konner and Eaton estimate that ancestral hunter-gatherers obtained 35 percent to 40 percent of total calories from carbohydrates. I've seen other estimates as low as 22 percent. Reality likely falls between 22 percent and 65 percent. When pressed for a brief answer as to how many carbohydrate calories are in the Paleo diet, I say, "about a third of the total." By comparison, the typical U.S. diet provides 50 percent of calories from carbohydrate.

Someone could end up with a high-carb Paleo diet easily, by emphasizing tubers (e.g., potatoes), higher-carb vegetables, fruits, berries, and nuts (especially cashews). Compared with the SAD, this could cause higher or lower blood sugars, or no net change.

Any person with diabetes making a change in diet should do it in consultation with a personal physician or other qualified healthcare professional familiar with their case.

Wanting to hear from women with diabetes who'd actually tested some of these specialty diets, I reached out to Catherine

Vancak. In her blog, *A Diabetic Ballerina*, she writes about her experiment with the Paleo diet.

- *Blood sugars are steady as a rock! I ate about 50 grams of carbs per day so my mealtime boluses were much smaller than what I was used to. By consuming less carbohydrates and taking less insulin, my lows and highs were smoothed out. Since I was also eating more fat (healthy fats, of course), any spikes I had were much slower. I still needed my basal and I made sure I bolused for every gram of carbohydrates, even veggies. All in all my blood sugars were almost normal. Wow!*
- *I realized that processed foods made me feel sick. On Paleo I made sure to eat foods that were minimally processed. I ate fresh fruits and veggies, organic meats, nuts and seeds without any seasoning. I played with recipes to create my own banana bread, brownies, egg muffins, and fritattas. The ingredients were so simple! For example my banana bread just contained ripe bananas, eggs, almond flour, almond butter, and vanilla! Once I had eaten these unprocessed foods for a while I realized that my body didn't feel achy and tired. It was a nice experience to get rid of the chemicals that I couldn't pronounce.*
- *I gained weight! I know it sounds funny but I actually gained weight eating Paleo! Since I was consuming a lot of healthy fat my blood sugars weren't too affected, so I thought "fats didn't count!" I am always conscious of the carbs that I eat but I forgot about fat and fat has lots of calories, too. I didn't gain too much weight but good to know!*
- *Feeling full and with lots of energy, I was able to dance and complete my workouts just as much as I was before I started eating Paleo. Even though my*

carbohydrate intake was low I didn't experience any dip in energy at all.

■ *I missed my favorite foods. I love cereal, I'm just going to be honest. I think restricting myself so much put my favorite foods even higher on the pedestal of things I wanted. For quite a while I didn't crave sugar or grains, but after a while I needed to have a little bit of my favorites to keep my sanity.*

■ *What did I learn and what will I take away from my Paleo test drive? The less carbohydrate equals less mealtime insulin equals smoothed out blood sugars. I'll definitely be keeping a close eye on my carbs. I also realized that processed foods make me feel like garbage. Even though I'm eating some crackers or cereal I'm going to make sure I can pronounce (and KNOW) what the ingredients are. Fats still have calories! Eating healthy fats like omega-3s helps keep me full and slows down my carbohydrate spikes, but overeating them isn't helpful either. Speaking of fats, I love coconut oil! I had never experienced it before I tried Paleo and it's great!*

■ *Will I continue with Paleo? While I've enjoyed my time exploring what Paleo has to offer me, I think that my original way of eating (balanced portion control) will be better for me to maintain in the long run. I have learned a lot and I'll be making a few adjustments. I'm definitely cutting out the processed food and keeping my carb intake low. It's still a work in progress for me to figure out a healthy, long-term way of eating that keeps my weight in check for dance, keeps my blood sugar stable, and gives me energy to power through my classes. In a few more months I'll let you know how my next experiment goes.*

Sysy Morales says the Paleo, the Atkins, and the Raw Food Diet all appealed to her because of the possibility of reducing insulin. "The less insulin I use, the easier it is for me to manage my blood sugars. I would like to lose some weight so I always hoped these diets would bring about that side effect, too.

"I eat a wide variety of foods. I try to eat intuitively, asking myself what I feel like eating. Sometimes I'll have grapefruit for breakfast or an egg, or almond butter on celery, or an avocado. Lunch is usually some kind of vegetable or salad and some fish, chicken, lamb, or beef. I do enjoy quinoa and legumes and eat small amounts of each. If I snack it's usually fruit, something low glycemic like cherries or blueberries. If I really want to indulge but not give in to cake or something like that, I'll have a bowl of cut-up mango or strawberries with whipped cream.

"I see this as a lifelong way of eating. Sometimes I will have champagne and chocolate for a special night with my husband but overall, I stick to this way of eating. It feels restrictive when I'm in a public setting where everyone is digging into ice cream and donuts; otherwise, at home, I feel very satisfied with the way I eat.

"In the summer, I feel best on a raw food diet because I tend to overheat easily and it seems to keep me cool and energetic. In the winter I do more Paleo/Atkins because [I]feel the need for more stews and meats and heavier, warming foods. It's challenging to eat an entirely raw food diet. Most people simply will not stick with it. The Atkins diet that people have come to know has been misinterpreted by media because only the initial stage of the diet is very-low carb. Past that stage, the Atkins diet is much like the Paleo diet. Whole foods are promoted and grains are to be eaten so long as one can manage their weight and blood sugars. These two diets are much easier to stick with because if you eat a lot of fruits and vegetables and sources of protein, the food choices are endless. I like combining the ideas of the Clean Diet with my mix of Paleo, Atkins, and the Raw Food diet to get something that is customized to me, personally."

Sysy's favorite meal is the French salad called Nicoise. Here is the recipe she follows for Nicoise salad:

1 grilled tuna steak or 2 cans of tuna
3 hard-boiled eggs, peeled and either halved or quartered
3 small new red potatoes, diced
Boston or butter lettuce
2–3 small ripe tomatoes, cored and cut into eighths
1 small red onion, sliced very thin
8 ounces green beans
1/4 cup olives
2 Tbsp capers, rinsed and/or several anchovies

Dressing
A blend of lemon juice, extra-virgin olive oil, minced shallots, a few shakes of fresh thyme,basil and oregano leaves, a dollop of Dijon mustard, and a sprinkle of salt and pepper.

Preparation
Marinate tuna steak in a little olive oil. Heat a large skillet on medium high heat, or place on a hot grill. Cook the steak 2 to 3 minutes on each side until cooked through.
Boil potatoes, add 1 tablespoon salt and cook until potatoes are tender, 5 to 8 minutes. Transfer potatoes to a medium bowl with a slotted spoon (do not discard boiling water). Toss warm potatoes with 1/4 cup vinaigrette; set aside.
While potatoes are cooking, toss lettuce with 1/4 cup vinaigrette in large bowl until coated. Arrange bed of lettuce on a serving platter, place tuna in center of lettuce. Toss tomatoes, red onion, 3 tablespoons vinaigrette, and salt and pepper to taste in bowl; arrange tomato-onion mixture on the lettuce bed. Arrange reserved potatoes in a mound at edge of lettuce bed.

Return water to boil; add 1 tablespoon salt and green beans. Cook until tender but crisp, 3 to 5 minutes. Drain beans, transfer to reserved ice water, and let stand until just cool, about 30 seconds; dry beans well. Toss beans, 3 tablespoons vinaigrette, and salt and pepper to taste; arrange in a mound at edge of lettuce bed.

Arrange hard boiled eggs, olives, and anchovies (if using) in mounds on the lettuce bed. Drizzle eggs with remaining 2 tablespoons dressing, sprinkle entire salad with capers (if using), and serve immediately.

Elizabeth Edelman of *Diabetes Daily* says she just ended her run with the Dukan diet, a low-carb, low-fat diet. "I would have continued but I got burned out eating only fat-free yogurt, eggs, and rotisserie chicken. So yes, I do find them difficult to maintain. Super low-carb diets are not something I can follow for the long term. Nor would I really want to. I believe that carbohydrates are vital to a healthy and balanced diet.

"When I was doing the Dukan diet, intense exercise was not encouraged. I have a daily yoga practice and in order to maintain that I need fuel. I always ate a banana before I did yoga, I need it for sustenance. I was always tired from doing low-carb also, so I upped my coffee intake when I was doing it. Probably not the best!"

Kelly Love Johnson started researching Paleo and clean eating about a year ago and says a lot of the research made sense. "I had pretty good control with my BG [blood glucose], but wanted it to be better. After my initial diagnosis, I really focused on limiting carb intake. That and giving up alcohol is likely responsible for the first 50 pounds I lost in 2005. I also 'tried' not to eat anything with HFCS [high fructose corn syrup]. I was better about HFCS in the beginning, but you probably know that it's in almost everything! My biggest challenge was convenience and the fact that I don't really cook (or enjoy cooking). But after reading a lot of info on Paleo and clean eating, I decided to start incorporating some changes in my eating plan. My former healthy plan was good—lots of veggies, fruit, etc., but even my salad dressing had HFCS. And I was reading some scary things about Splenda (which I used to put in everything). I also ate low-carb or sugar-free convenience foods—pudding snacks, gelatin—and I started to think seriously about the chemicals I was putting in my body every day."

Kelly doesn't adhere strictly to Paleo. "I'm not gluten free and I won't eat pork. I can't give up dairy (won't) or artificial sweeteners, though I do stick to Stevia now (or agave or honey). I did switch to organic dairy products 100 percent, along with organic meats. One of the reasons I don't adhere strictly to Paleo is that I just can't eat that much meat. I eat chicken (organic) two or three times a week, fish (usually Alaskan salmon or light tuna in water—not albacore, because it's been shown to be higher in mercury). It doesn't feel restrictive because I always have more than enough to eat (and I'm not counting net carbs every meal). I gave up processed sugar which is even in 'healthy' foods (I recently discovered that my favorite Wasa cracker has it, but they have three other flavors that do not have sugar and I'm eating those now). I read labels in a different way now ... actually, I read fewer labels because I'm eating very little processed food. I buy a lot of food in the bulk section of the grocery store now: beans, barley, quinoa. On a typical day I'll have Greek yogurt (2 percent) or oatmeal (with a little milk) because I find if I eat a little fat with breakfast I don't get hungry before lunchtime. This is my biggest challenge. I've always been a coffee for breakfast person and that's definitely not good for BG control. I try to redefine what breakfast is."

Breakfast: "This morning I had half of a sliced avocado and four Wasa fiber crackers. People don't usually think of avocado for breakfast, but it works for me. Healthy fats (walnuts, olive oil, avocado) are definitely a Paleo choice."

Lunch: "I most often have what was leftover from the night before … chicken breast and spinach with garlic, sliced organic tomatoes, and so on."

Dinner: "I put a lot of thought into dinner because I still don't love to cook (it's starting to grow on me, though) and I try to cook every third night if I can. I just made a big pot of quinoa salad with dried cranberries, walnuts, green onion, mint, and garbanzo beans. I'll have that for dinner tonight. Tomorrow I'll take it for lunch. Tomorrow night I'll mix it up with baked organic chicken breast and throw in some Clementine orange sections and heat it up. I make Kasha (buckwheat groats) with chicken stock (I'll buy organic boxed because I'm never organized enough to make my own) and it will literally be good for three or four meals. I have to change it up though, throw a hard-boiled egg in and eat some for breakfast, mix it with sunflower seeds and dried cranberries for a snack, and so on."

Snacks: "I snack on walnuts, almonds, pecans, dried fruit (from the bulk section, not the prebagged, sugar-added kind). I love goat cheese and the stores here carry spreadable organic goat cheese as 'breakfast cheese' I put it on Wasa whole grain for a snack or lunch. I eat organic cottage cheese, and put organic milk in my coffee. I can't give up coffee either, but I do switch to green tea at the office and drink green or roobios tea all day."

Kelly's perspective of eating right has changed since her diagnosis. "I'll never look at eating as a "diet" or short term plan. I do think it's sustainable over the long term if you can gradually replace what's in your pantry now with unprocessed food. I didn't throw my wheat pasta, soba noodles, and sugar-free pudding away one day. I just started incorporating new things as I did research and read about Paleo and clean eating. Chemical free is the goal and that really simplifies things for me. The hardest thing is eating out! I try to choose restaurants that I feel comfortable asking 'Can you do this or that?' (no fast food, obviously, but I gave that up years ago … except for Wendy's salads, and I gave those up last year). I love sushi restaurants because you can get sashimi or sushi with brown rice and it's super healthy and high in protein if you stay away from anything fried or the sushi rolls with cream cheese. I'm also lucky that healthy restaurants are not hard to find at all in Austin. Also, I do have weeks where I'm like 'Ugh, I absolutely cannot cook this week!' There's a place here called My Fit Foods and they have great, reasonably priced pre-made meals, no preservatives, never frozen, about 80 percent would fit into Paleo, 100 percent clean eating. I'll order three or four days' worth, pick it up, and it's always more than I need, plus, I get a break from cooking. I don't feel deprived at all, but I do wake up hungry. I've learned that waking up hungry is a sign that your metabolism is working as it should!"

Kelly says the benefits of the Paleo diet have also included better sleep. "I don't have insomnia anymore (knock wood). I'm amazed that I don't want to hit the snooze button 15 times in the morning, or that I can close my eyes at 10:00 p.m. and actually fall asleep. I have gradually eliminated chemicals from my food over the past nine or ten months and I can only explain it by saying my body feels like it's working as it should. I definitely have better BG control. My last A1C was five-point-something. I've had as good before, but have seen them climb to seven-point-something gradually over the past two years, which is when doctors tend to want to add a second medication and I wanted to avoid that— and if possible, get off of metformin! I feel like these changes were a good way to reinforce healthy habits. There are some Paleo recipes I like, mostly things like quinoa salads (but I tend to do my own twist once I've made something once or twice). I find more recipes that suit me on clean eating sites—I really like cleaneatingmag.com. They break it down 'quick and easy' (yes), '20 minutes or less' (yes), 'budget' (yes!). They also have printable meal plans and recipe lists. My go-to super fast and easy are sweet potato fries, and I used to make them from scratch, but then I found an organic brand in the freezer section—no chemicals, no preservatives—and they're great to have on hand to throw in the oven for a quick meal."

AUTHENTIC ADVICE

■ *I probably eat half of the protein that your average person on Paleo eats, mostly because I don't love meat and I don't care for tofu. But my changes are definitely Paleo inspired in that the goal is to eat unprocessed back to basics food. I love going to farmer's markets and they have several here all year round. I can buy goat cheese and milk from the farmer who owns the goats. I can buy fresh eggs, vegetables that have never been in a store, artisan and local olive oil, balsamic vinegar, and honey. I'm definitely an advocate for eating as locally as you can! Final tip: There are some "paleo" and "clean eating" web sites that claim their eating plan can "cure" diabetes. There is no cure for diabetes, even type 2 diabetes. There is control and management, but there is currently no cure.* ■ Kelly Love Johnson

■ *I would advise others to try an eating plan after researching it properly. Be careful with the Atkins diet if you don't like vegetables because you will be very limited to animal protein sources and that can be uncomfortable and unhealthy and difficult to sustain. When trying a new diet, keep a food journal so you can write about your moods and energy levels and reactions to the foods you eat. Don't be afraid to customize a diet for yourself. We all have different needs and experimenting with different foods should be something we all do to find the right mix for us.* ■ Sysy Morales

4   The Carbohydrate: Good? Bad? Less or More?

My favorite food in the world used to be breakfast cereal. I loved Golden Grahams, Cinnamon Life, Oatmeal Squares, and all types of granola. I tried to pick the lower carbs brands, the ones that have 25 to 27 carbs per serving, but my blood sugar spiked and then dropped no matter how much insulin I injected. I refused for years to give up my morning routine because the thought of eggs for breakfast made me want to gag. I lived with the roller-coaster spike and fall of my blood sugars for years until I became pregnant for the first time and finally said goodbye to breakfast cereal. I was sad and mad at diabetes, but my blood sugars were much improved.

Today I eat an egg omelet with ham and cheese with sautéed kale for breakfast every morning and it's delicious. Sometimes I'll add a whole wheat English muffin or wrap the omelet in a whole wheat tortilla, but that's the exception, not the norm. Looking back, it's hard to believe I went for so long eating such a high carb breakfast. I've learned a lot about fueling my body through writing this book and talking to the various experts, and in this chapter I'll share what I've learned about carbohydrates.

Carbohydrates have become the ugly step sister in the family photo album of healthy eating. Standing in the grocery aisle, consumers study ingredients and food labels, counting and analyzing the carb content of their foods. In the last decade, the popularity of low-carb diets rose to dramatic heights as Americans gravitated toward the South Beach, Atkins, and Zone diets. Fruits were forsaken for plates piled high with steak and eggs.

People with diabetes have been counting carbs for years, and many adhere passionately to the philosophy of doctors like Dr. Bernstein, whose advice (6 grams of carbs for breakfast, 12 at lunch and dinner) differs from the Academy of Nutrition and Dietetics (AND) recommendations (45–60 grams per meal) for a healthy diet. But something gets lost in the fervor over carbohydrates, and that is the reality that even ugly stepsisters have redeeming qualities.

There are two basic types of carbohydrates: simple or "bad" and complex or "good."

"Good" carbs are found in some of the following:

- Oatmeal, oat bran
- Nuts and seeds
- Most fruits (e.g., strawberries, blueberries, pears, and apples)
- Most vegetables
- Dry beans and peas
- Whole wheat bread, wheat bran
- Barley, brown rice, couscous, bulgur or whole grain cereals

"Bad" carbs include sugars found naturally in foods such as fruits, vegetables, milk, and milk products. Simple carbohydrates also include sugars added during food processing and refining and include some of the following:

- Refined grains like white bread and white rice
- Processed foods such as cake, cookies, chips, certain lunch meats, hot dogs
- Soft drinks and certain types of alcohols, such as beer and wine.

I interviewed author and *Huffington Post* blogger Riva Greenberg for a controversial story in *Diabetes Health*. Conversations about carbs always seem to get people fired up, so this is not unusual. Greenberg has lived with type 1 diabetes since 1972 and says she used to think she ate a fairly low-carb diet. After graduating college and moving back to her native New York City, Greenberg ate the standard New York diet of bagels, muffins, scones, and pretzels, and it wasn't until she read Dr. Bernstein's *Diabetes Solution* that she began to change the way she ate. She gave up the bagels and pretzels, but took liberties with the rigid Bernstein diet. She continued to read the latest research on various meal plans, and had an "ah-ha!" moment when she realized she was using the term "low carb" incorrectly. "I thought I was eating a low-carb diet, but every day oatmeal, veggies, fruit, nuts, and beans make up the bulk of my diet and those all have carbs in them." Greenberg realized she was following a higher carb diet than she thought, yet it was low GI, and it was working.

Riva says routine helps. "If you can eat the same way most days, your blood sugars are more predictable." Most days her meals consist of the following:

Breakfast: Steel-cut oatmeal with flaxseed, sunflower seeds, berries, a spoonful of nonfat Greek yogurt and cottage cheese and peanut butter

Lunch: Leftover veggies, chick peas, and turkey, chicken, hummus or feta cheese

Dinner: Chicken or fish, nonstarchy vegetables, beans, and a glass of red wine

Snacks: Dark chocolate, fruit and nuts

"I'm not saying I never eat pancakes, fried calamari, or the occasional dessert, and I do always dunk the bread crusts in olive oil when I'm out to dinner. But pretty much the way I eat now is simple and really clean," she says. "Eating this way I've been able to maintain my lowest weight without much effort. I also don't feel deprived. I like what I eat. I don't miss bagels at all." Greenberg believes that when you change your eating habits, over time your taste buds change. "I also think that when you shift your mindset from feeling deprived to wanting to be healthy, then it doesn't feel like giving up processed foods and refined carbohydrates is a sacrifice."

Michelle Sorensen agrees and says, "I think I have gradually become aware of how lower GI foods help stabilize my blood sugar levels and that all the 'white stuff' is not very good for me. I will still have white rice at times, but try to use quinoa or brown rice instead. However, eating better carbs is not just about managing diabetes for me ... it is about overall health. I know that when I used to eat a lot of pasta and bread before going gluten free, I had a good A1C at times, but I was tired and sluggish, my moods were less stable, and I had symptoms of candida in my system. Now I look to get all my carbs and protein from healthy sources that provide nutrition rather than empty calories."

Food is a complex issue for people with diabetes. What we eat effects how we feel, physically and emotionally. Everyone is different, and what works for one may not work for another. What's most important when making food choices is to be informed, know the difference between good and bad carbs, and choose what works best for you.

What about low-carb diets? Researchers continue to investigate low-carbohydrate, high-protein diets in people with diabetes. A review of thirteen studies found that low-carbohydrate diets consistently lower levels of hemoglobin A1C, a test that measures blood glucose control over the previous two to three months, and triglycerides, a type of fat in the blood, in people with diabetes.

For weight loss, however, the review found that low-carb diets are no more effective than regimens that limit fat intake. The American Diabetes Association has stated that both low-fat and low-carbohydrate diets may be effective for up to one year, but it's most important to find a healthy, weight-management diet you can stick with.

THE JOHNS HOPKINS HEALTH ALERT STATES THAT ...

The American Diabetes Association recommends that 45 percent to 65 percent of your total calories come from carbohydrates. This may sound counterproductive, since people with diabetes need to control their blood glucose levels. However, carbohydrates are an important source of energy, water-soluble vitamins, minerals, and fiber, so restricting total carbohydrate intake to less than 130 grams per day is not recommended. In addition, some experts have relaxed the allowance for ordinary sugar intake to as much as 10 percent of total calories. That means that people with diabetes can have a limited amount of sweets, chocolates, and desserts as part of a healthy meal plan.

It's worth noting that the long-term effects of extreme low-carbohydrate diets are not known. What's more, many doctors are concerned that low-carbohydrate intake may cause ketosis and that high protein intake can damage the heart and the kidneys—all of which are already risks for people with diabetes. Studies have shown that people who have diabetes and chronic kidney disease may help prevent further damage to their kidneys by reducing the amount of protein in their diet. The American Diabetes Association does not recommend low-carbohydrate diets for the management of diabetes.

On her *Diabetes Self-Management* blog, Tara Dairman reported:

On Friday, December 28, the American Diabetes Association (ADA) issued its 2008 Clinical Practice Recommendations, which are a set of guidelines that help health-care providers treat people with diabetes based on the most current scientific evidence. One key change in this year's recommendations is the inclusion of low-carbohydrate diets as an option for people with diabetes who are trying to lose weight.

According to the "Medical Nutrition Therapy" section of the new guidelines, "either low-carbohydrate or low-fat calorie-restricted diets may be effective in the short-term (up to one year)" for weight loss in people with diabetes. This statement represents a significant reversal from the ADA's former position on low-carbohydrate diets. For instance, the agency's 2007 recommendations stated that such diets were not recommended for the treatment of overweight/obesity—even in the short term—because their long-term effects were unknown and they did not seem to provide better maintenance of weight loss than low-fat diets over the long term. But in a press release that accompanied the publication of the 2008 recommendations, the ADA has stated that "there is now evidence that the most important determinant of weight loss is not the composition of the diet, but whether the person can stick with it, and that some individuals are more likely to adhere to a low carbohydrate diet while others may find a low fat calorie-restricted diet easier to follow."

In the same press release, ADA President of Health Care & Education Ann Albright, Ph.D., R.D., stated "We're not endorsing either of these weight-loss plans over any other method of losing weight." More important, she said, is that people with diabetes choose a weight-loss plan that works for them, and that their health-care team supports their efforts and monitors their health accordingly.

Indeed, the ADA's new guidelines lay out specific instructions for monitoring the health of people who are on low-carbohydrate diets. Because people following these eating plans may replace calories from carbohydrate with fat or protein, the ADA recommends that health-care providers monitor their lipid profiles (including cholesterol and triglyceride levels). Because extra protein in the diet may make kidney problems worse, the ADA also recommends that people with nephropathy have their kidney function monitored and be counseled about including the correct amount of protein in their diets. Finally, the new recommendations point out that providers may need to adjust the blood-glucose–lowering drug therapy of people who reduce their carbohydrate intake.

The "low-carb vs. low-fat" diet debate has been raging in the diabetes community for some time. On our own blog, David Spero addressed the issue in his post "Carbs vs. Fats—Who's to Blame?" There he argued in favor of low-carbohydrate diets, and many readers shared comments detailing their own experiences with them. Jan Chait, who favors the low-fat approach for her needs, responded with her own post on the subject, "Fitting Diabetes Into Your Lifestyle." The ADA's revised recommendations reflect the growing evidence that either approach, combined with regular physical activity, can be an effective choice for those who need to lose weight.

Some other changes present in this year's Clinical Practice Recommendations include new guidelines on maintaining a diabetes "disaster kit" to be used in case of emergency; revisions and additions to treatment recommendations for older adults with diabetes and children and adolescents with type 1 diabetes; a new section on type 1 diabetes and hypothyroidism; and new emphasis on statin drug treatment for lipid level management and ACE inhibitor or ARB drug treatment to treat high blood pressure and nephropathy.

The American Diabetes Association's full annual Clinical Practice Recommendations were published in a supplement to the January 2008 issue of the journal *Diabetes Care*. You can find a summary of the revisions to the Clinical Practice Recommendations at:

http://care.diabetesjournals.org/content/31/Supplement_1/S3.full

And a summary of the full "Standards of Medical Care in Diabetes—2008:

http://care.diabetesjournals.org/content/31/Supplement_1/S5.full

According to *Diabetes in Control*, a weekly newsletter for medical professionals, the American Diabetes Association's announcement is a breakthrough because the group is the first major health organization to give any support to low-carb diets. Mary Vernon, MD, CMD, chairman of the board of the American Society of Bariatric Physicians, and author of *Atkins Diabetes Revolution* (Morrow, 2004) stated that, "We're pleased that they're willing to move away from an entrenched position and look at the science. But it's not enough and it isn't respectful enough of how effective this is as a change in patients." Vernon would like to see more recommendations about patient monitoring and continuing education for physicians. "Most doctors aren't familiar with using this technique because they've been told not to do it up until now," she said. "You have to be educated about how to use it." She warned that people with diabetes could experience bad outcomes if their doctors don't have the right information. "If you drop your carbs and don't change your medication, it's very likely you'll have too much medicine for your body and you'll have side effects," she said. "Then the diet gets blamed when it's not the diet's fault at all."

Vernon would also like to see the American Diabetes Association back off their restriction that people stay on low-carb diets for no more than a year. "What happens if, after a year, your blood sugars are good—should you quit?" she said. "We don't take people off their medicine if it's working. It's not fair to hold this diet to a standard that nothing else is held to."

Rachel Garlinghouse does not follow the American Diabetes Association's diet. "For one, diabetes is such a personal, individual disease. One diet can in no way fit 'all.' A recent book entitled *Sugar Nation* by Jeff O'Connell really changed the way I looked at eating with diabetes. The idea that a diabetic can basically eat whatever he or she wants as long as it's covered by insulin is killing us. Although I didn't eliminate most carbohydrates as the book's author suggested, I am working hard to eat more protein and less carbs. As the author talks about in his book, no one tells a person who is lactose intolerant to consume lactose, so why do the ADA and diabetes professionals not tell diabetics to drastically reduce carbs, which cause sugar spikes? Truly, I believe it's time for medical professionals to stop pacifying diabetics and the public. What we are eating, how we eat, and our lack of exercise is killing us. There needs to be drastic changes made to the American diet."

A Typical Meal Plan from Rachel Garlinghouse:

Breakfast: "A glass of water and a bowl of oatmeal made with milk."
Lunch: "Leftovers from the evening before."
Dinner: "A homemade, vegetarian, organic meal—usually soup and homemade whole wheat bread, low-carb pasta with tofu, veggies, cheese, and sauce, stir fry with edamame, veggies, and tofu, or, if I need something quick, scrambled eggs, sweet potato fries, and a tangerine."
Afternoon snack: "Greek yogurt mixed with fruit puree (no sugar added)."

"My husband and I eat dessert together every night before bed. The dessert is always something homemade such as my current favorite, Scottish shortbread made with almond flour and drizzled with dark chocolate."

Elizabeth Edelman, Chief Executive Officer, *Diabetes Daily* says, "I love carbs. They are delicious. As a girl with French and Italian blood, carbs are a part of my genetic makeup. Because of my diabetes, it is difficult for me to enjoy them with abandon as I once did in my youth. Nowadays, I stick to a modified version of a low-carb diet. I do this for two reasons: One, I find it much easier to control my blood sugar levels when I cut out things like bread and pasta. Two, I do it for weight management. I was vegan for a good chunk of last year and packed on almost fifteen pounds onto my 5 foot 2 inch frame switching to a more carb heavy plant based diet. Counting carbs is like second nature to most people who live with diabetes. I learned from a really wonderful dietitian after my diagnosis. I am not perfect at it 100 percent of the time, but I feel that I have a pretty good grasp on it. I do little modifications to help me not go too overboard in situations like going out to eat.

When I am at a restaurant, I typically order a salad with protein or something similar to help minimize the guesswork of hidden carbs. Doing little things like that pays dividends when you don't have the inevitable blood sugar spike from hidden carbohydrates in restaurant food."

Meagan Esler also loves carbs and says, "If it was allowed, I might just marry a cupcake. Though, we'd likely have a dysfunctional relationship because carbs and I don't get along as well as I'd like. When I restrict them too much I feel sick, when I eat too many I also feel sick and sometimes end up dealing with elevated blood sugars.

"Even though I live in Chicago, one of the best places around for getting amazing pizza, pizza is one of my rare foods because of the unfriendly high carb count and fat content. My blood sugars go up and sometimes even require more than one insulin shot when I eat pizza. Because of this, my husband and I created our own recipe for 'Pizza Sausage Soup' since we could incorporate the flavors of all our favorite pizza ingredients in a soup that has an extremely low carb count. Instead of pizza crust, most of the carbohydrates in this soup come from healthy, fiber-filled cannellini beans, and yes, we top it off with gooey, cheesy mozzarella.

"I don't follow an extremely low-carb diet because if I did, I'm afraid I'd run out in a panic and go crazy in a pastry shop. I try to enjoy my carbs in moderation. This keeps me from going nuts, feeling sick, or feeling deprived. My body is happy, my blood sugars are happy, and I find I can stick to this way of eating."

Michelle Sorensen says her diet has evolved over her twelve years with diabetes, and has become plant-based and 99 percent vegan. "I have definitely noticed that my A1C is better when I am eating less simple carbs and more complex carbs from vegetables, whole grains, and legumes. Even more important than the A1C result is that I have high and low fluctuations. I find that if I need less insulin for my meals then there is less likelihood of spiking really high or dropping really low. I may not always get my dose of insulin right, but if I am taking 2 units I am less likely to make a serious error than when I need 4 or 5 units."

Franziska Spritzler, RD, CDE, says she counts carbs at every meal. "I don't use the exchange system, but I do count carbs using ADA exchange lists and food labels. I'm a CDE, so I've taught many patients to count carbs as well. I do not follow ADA guidelines regarding Create Your Plate with 45 to 60 grams of carbs per meal; that amount of carbs is closer to what I eat for the entire day. I typically eat 15 to 20 grams of carbs per meal, closer to 20 grams most of the time. I count net carbs, subtracting fiber from the total carb count." Franziska's diet is lower than ADA recommendations, yet not as strict as Dr. Bernstein's. "I generally do not snack. This way of eating works well for me. I rarely get hungry, and I can still eat things like fruit, yams, and winter squash in moderation while keeping my blood sugar under control."

Typical Intake for Franziska:

Breakfast: "Four ounces. sardines/salmon OR 2 eggs with 2 cups kale or spinach cooked in 1 tablespoon butter or coconut oil; 1/2 cup fruit OR 1/2 cup sweet potato, 2 Brazil nuts, and green tea."

Lunch: "Usually leftovers from dinner (same amount) OR 1 cup plain Greek yogurt, 2 cups chopped raw vegetables, 4 olives, and 3 tablespoons guacamole; 1/2 cup fruit, 1 tablespoon almond butter with small square of dark chocolate, and water."

Dinner: "Four ounces. beef/fish/poultry, 2–3 cups raw or cooked non starchy vegetables with 2 tablespoons olive oil, 1/2 cup sweet potato OR fruit, 1 tablespoon almond butter, and water."

"I'm a committed low-carber. Following the ADA [American Diabetes Association] plan would result in excessive glucose excursions for me because I am not on insulin or oral meds," says Franziska.

People with diabetes have been counting carbs for years, and many adhere passionately to the philosophy of doctors like Dr. Bernstein, whose advice differs from the ADA, in that he recommends a lower carb intake for a healthy diet. He has a lot of passionate followers, as do the Dukan diet, the Mayo Clinic diet, the Vegan diet, and the Atkins diet, among others. On the website she co-founded with her husband David www.*DiabetesDaily*.com, Elizabeth Edelman writes about experimenting with the low-carb Dukan diet.

A while back, I began Weight Watchers to lose a few pounds that I put on from a high carbohydrate, vegan diet. I lost a few pounds, and coupled with the running I have been doing, my weight is almost back to normal. Then the holidays hit. And while I don't feel I have put on too much extra, I am definitely a little more snug in my clothes than I was a week or two ago.

I was scouring Amazon for some interesting diet books and came across the Dukan diet. Apparently, Princess Kate is on this diet, and although I think she could stand to eat a sandwich, or 50 ... it looks like the celebrities are picking this book up and when that happens it is sure to catch on to mainstream America.

So what is the Dukan diet? It is another form of a low-carbohydrate diet. Except there are some noticeable differences that I can see just from the first couple chapters that sets it apart from the other low-carb diets out there. Dr. Pierre Dukan has worked with many overweight people in all walks of life to help them find a permanent solution to their weight-loss endeavors. Permanent you say? I'd like to see that in practice!

How is it different from say, Atkins, South Beach, or Bernstein? *Dukan has four phases of the diet to get you to where you want to be. The first phase is called the Attack Phase. For 2 to 7 days, the only thing that you eat is pure protein. No fruits, no veggies— only lean meats, fish, low-fat dairy, and lots and lots and lots of water. Just less than 2 quarts. Yes, diet soda is allowed, and even encouraged! You also eat 1-1/2 tablespoons of oat bran per day to help you feel full and staying regular.*

The next phase is called the Cruise Phase. *Here, you begin to add some vegetables in with your protein—every other day until you reach your goal. Vegetables allowed are ones that we as diabetics are encouraged to eat: tomatoes, cucumbers, radishes, spinach, asparagus, leeks, green beans, cabbage, mush-rooms, celery, fennel, lettuce of all kinds, eggplant, zucchini, summer squash, and peppers. Avoid starchy veggies like potatoes, corn, peas, beans, or lentils. But we already know those have carbohydrates.*

After the Cruise Phase is successfully completed, you begin the Consolidation Phase. *In this much less restrictive phase, you add fruits back in to your diet as well as bread, cheese, and the other more starchy vegetables. You stay on this phase for 5 days for every pound lost. You also pick one day a week where you go back to the pure protein Attack Phase, and do it every week.*

Finally, you reach the last phase: Stabilization. *You are able to eat what you like but only following* *these three rules: Go back to the Attack Phase one day a week, every week, for the rest of your life, No more elevators or escalators. And finally—tablespoons of oat bran every day for the rest of your life. Manage-able? Let's see!*

I am not a big fan of the low-carb diet. If you know who I am, I love my carbs and I love that, if you choose them correctly, they are an integral part of a healthy diet. However, I do like to see what the big fuss from all of these diets is about also. I am going to try the Dukan diet out and see how I like it. I'm going to monitor my weight loss here, on Diabetes Daily. I am going to talk about how the diet is affecting my health, which I can monitor at my endocrinologist's office. And I am going to see if this is something that I can adopt as a lifestyle. As a former vegan, I am a little wary of pure protein days ... but I think I will be okay once I see the results. Will there be a change in my A1C for the better? Will these 5 pounds finally go away once and for all? Will I become a low-carb believer? Stay tuned to find out!

I followed up with Elizabeth who said she just ended her run with the Dukan diet. "I understand the hype surrounding low-carb diets. They provide quick results if you're trying to lose weight and are typically easy to maintain if you're into eating meat all the time. They are also a good way to help your blood sugar levels to stabilize. Low carbs is less insulin which is less room for error. The two weeks I was on the Dukan diet my Dexcom showed an essentially flat line. I was amazed. But I was hungry for a croissant." Elizabeth says she typically eats at most 25 grams per meal and leaves 25 grams for snacks throughout the day. "I find that works best for me, giving me the variety of foods I enjoy while still allowing for weight loss/ maintenance."

Elizabeth's Typical Meals Consist of:

- *Breakfast:* "A whole grapefruit and two pieces of turkey bacon or a hard boiled egg."
- *Snack:* "String cheese, nuts, yogurt, and celery with peanut butter or hummus throughout the day."
- *Lunch:* "A salad, with balsamic dressing I make at home, or soup."
- *Dinner:* "A piece of fish, chicken, or the occasional steak, and two kinds of veggies or a salad."

"I also enjoy coffee with milk and lots of water throughout the day. If I want *dessert,* I eat a piece of fruit (Clementines are my fave right now) or some chocolate covered almonds. I am also a Jeni's ice cream addict, and I buy these teeny tiny ice cream cones for my daughter—they hold like two tablespoons of ice cream. So I indulge every now and then. I make sure it's real food, though, so my craving is satisfied and I don't over do it."

Elizabeth says, "As far as I'm concerned, there is no such thing as a bad carb .... Just kidding. Any carb can be a challenge when you're eating with diabetes. However, when I eat carbs I stick to whole grains. I don't do white rice or white bread. When I eat them I always opt for brown rice and whole wheat bread. I also make sure that if I am eating something carb heavy that it's not something that's fried, too. Another thing I look for when I eat carbs is fiber. I love fruit, which is packed with fiber. Whole grains, too."

Michelle Sorensen agrees and says, "I would never follow a Dr. Bernstein diet because I eat vegan and gluten free. I'm not sure I would want to stick to a specific carb count for each meal. I would rather match my insulin to the amount of carbs I eat, and expect that number to vary depending on my level of activity and what food I have available to eat."

Fransizka says she's found it pretty easy to follow a low-carb diet. "Truly, nothing is off limits as long as I eat very small portions of high-carb foods. Eating higher amounts of fat and protein keep me satisfied, and I experience reactive hypoglycemia less often and less severely than when I was eating more carbohydrates. I definitely feel that I can keep my blood sugar under better control by low carbing. The fewer carbs I eat, the less my blood sugars rise, and the less insulin I need. By limiting carbs, I hope to preserve as much beta cell function as possible."

Sysy Morales doesn't follow a strict Dr. Bernstein-type of diet, "but his Law of Small Numbers is scientifically correct and has made a huge impact on my life and diabetes management. I eat 15 to 30 carbs per meal on most days and find that it's the only way for me to keep my blood sugars near non-diabetic range as well as avoid sharp lows and highs. I don't thrive on a high-fat diet, if I did I'd eat more like Dr. Bernstein. Since I don't, I increase my carb amount. For me and my diabetes management, good carbs are classified as any carbs that are not derived from processed foods. I do not view potatoes as bad carbs, for example. I see them as a healthy food that some people can get away with eating and some cannot. I eat them as a treat every now and then. I can eat sweet potatoes more often because they have a lower glycemic index [GI] than white potatoes. That's how I use the GI."

Sysy loves fish, but gets easily intimidated about how to cook it. "That is until I found out about poaching it. My favorite recipe is taking either tilapia or salmon filets and placing them on foil or in a shallow oven-proof glass container, coating them with salt and pepper, and topping with lemon and parsley. Then I add white wine (pinot grigio or sauvignon blanc) to cover the filets. I fold up the edges of the foil so that it becomes kind of like a bowl for the fish and wine or I cover the glass container with foil and then I cook in the oven at 400 to 425 degrees for 15 to 25 minutes, depending on the thickness of the fish, and viola!"

Baked Salmon Filets

1 pound salmon fillet, cut into four pieces
2 tablespoons dry white wine
1/4 teaspoon salt
Freshly ground pepper, to taste
2 tablespoons finely chopped shallot
Lemon wedges, for garnish

Preparation
Preheat oven to 425°F. Coat a 9-inch glass pie pan or an
   8-inch glass baking dish with cooking spray.
Place salmon, skin-side down, in the prepared pan. Sprinkle
   with wine.
Season with salt and pepper, then sprinkle with shallots.
   Cover with foil and bake until opaque in the center and
   starting to flake, 15 to 25 minutes, depending on thickness.
Spoon any liquid remaining in the pan over the salmon and
   serve with lemon wedges.

Rachel Garlinghouse has never followed a specific diet. "I try to eat a balanced and healthy amount of carbohydrates with each meal. The amount of carbs I eat at each meal can vary from meal to meal quite a bit depending on my blood sugar control that day, and what I'm craving. I don't look at food in terms of just the carbs and if they are good or bad. I simply live a healthy lifestyle that includes lots of healthy foods—whole grains, organic produce, fruits and veggies, homemade desserts made with lots of healthy ingredients, lean protein. I think when we start labeling carbs as good and bad, we walk a dangerous road. Because I often see very overweight people eating "good" foods—foods that claim to be low fat, high fiber, etc.—so people think they can eat all they want of these foods. The best way to avoid the ups and downs of dieting is not to diet at all, but to normalize a healthy lifestyle."

GOOD CARBS VS. BAD CARBS

Is there really any such thing as a good carb? As someone who has always loved carbs, it's been hard for me to wean myself off my high carbohydrate diet. I've lived with diabetes for nearly three decades, yet none of the medical professionals in my life ever encouraged me to change the way I ate. As long as my A1C was okay, and most of the time it was, no one suggested I eat eggs instead of cereal for breakfast or whole wheat instead of regular pasta. Of course, I've got plenty of food-related issues and sensitivities and maybe people tried to suggest alternate diets in subtle ways that I refused to hear. It's entirely possible. As a woman with diabetes I am very private and sensitive about what I put in my mouth and it's taken me nearly three decades to slowly change my eating habits. What I'm learning is that there are good and bad carbs, or to talk about it in a way that is not win/lose, there are carbs like sweet potatoes that don't require a lot of insulin. Education is an ongoing process and we can't do it alone.

Franziska says, "Before I discovered I had prediabetes/early diabetes, I wasn't sure that the glycemic index was valid. It seemed to me that as long as a meal contained protein and fat, the total carb amount would determine how much blood sugar would rise postprandially. However, once I began testing my own blood sugar an hour after eating, I realized that high GI foods like potatoes caused a significantly greater spike than an equal amount of carbohydrate from fruit or sweet potatoes. Even a piece of chocolate has less of an impact than potatoes or white rice. I believe this is because starch is comprised of glucose molecules alone, while fruit and table sugar contain both glucose and fructose. Fructose is metabolized differently and has a much lower GI than glucose: 19 vs. 100, respectively."

Rachel adds, "I do know about the glycemic index, and I believe that some foods are kinder to my blood sugars, such as brown rice, Dreamfields pasta, certain fruits, etc. I don't think the GI is a one-size-fits-all as each diabetic is different."

Much of the debate around low-carbohydrate eating is focused on the sustainability of a low-carb eating plan. Like Elizabeth Edelman said, rotisserie chicken got old and the Dukan diet was hard to maintain.

Rachel says, "One and a half weeks out of every month (pre-period and during my period weeks) my sugars skyrocket like clockwork. I ramp up the insulin, watch what I eat, sleep more, but it never fails that I struggle a lot during that time. A low-carb diet helps, but it by no means cures my issues. Do I think it's possible to stick to a low-carb diet for a lifetime? I love carbs—especially healthy desserts and fruits. I cannot imagine living low-carb all the time, to be honest. I think it is ideal for a diabetic to eat low-carb, because carbs are one cause of blood sugar issues. They cause ups and downs, even with proper insulin dosages. Will I ever go low-carb? I doubt it. I wish I could, but I have to be realistic."

Sysy believes the low-carb way of eating is sustainable because she is proof positive. "I've been able to sustain it and I'm a carb lover. However, I don't go too low in carbs, because then I need fat to get adequate calories and I don't feel well with more than a little fat in my diet. My husband doesn't have diabetes but he thrives on a high-fat and protein diet. Pasta, potatoes, desserts, all put him to sleep. Whereas steak and salad with a lot of olive oil makes him feel great."

Exercise is an important factor to consider when following a low-carb eating plan. Carbs are a great source of energy to get you going and help you maintain during your workouts.

Franziska says, "I walk at least an hour every day, typically one to two hours after eating, when my sugar is highest. My fuel comes from carbs, protein, and fat. I don't engage in anything more strenuous than walking and occasionally yoga or Pilates—again, always an hour or so after I eat in order to prevent hypoglycemia."

Sysy says, "I feel like I have enough energy for exercise and try to do it at least five days a week for an hour at a time. On the weekends my kids keep me busy so I'm still active. I think my fuel comes from foods like eggs, which have protein and fat, vegetables, and the small amounts of fruit I eat."

EXPERT ADVICE

Dr. Sheri Colberg-Ochs, exercise physiologist, professor of exercise science at Old Dominion University in Norfolk, Virginia, and a woman with type 1 diabetes, says "As long as a diet is isocaloric, meaning that you're eating enough to replace all the calories you use up in training, you can get by with as little as 40 percent of calories coming from carbs."

The study, "Glycaemic control, muscle glycogen and exercise performance in IDDM athletes on diets of varying carbohydrate content," found that high carbohydrate diets for athletes with diabetes worsened their blood sugar control, "These data do not support recommendations for IDDM athletes to consume a high carbohydrate diet, at least not when glycemic control worsens upon following this advice, as was observed in this short-term study."

In a *Diabetes Life* column, "Low Carb Eating and Exercise, Is Performance Compromised by Menu Choice?," Colberg-Ochs writes,

> *I have had many people ask me recently if they can follow a low-carb diet and still do significant exercise training and events—individuals with both type 1 and type 2 diabetes. Not all of us follow the "low-carb" mantra, but enough people do so that it's an issue that needs clarification. I'm not a carb advocate per se, but I realize the effect that carbs in moderation can have on performance. In spite of your body's improved use of fat and ketones on a low-carb regimen, fat will never be your body's first choice of fuels during moderate and intense workouts lasting more than a couple of minutes. If carbs are available, your body will use them over fats, especially as your workout gets more*

intense. It's simply because using carbs is more fuel efficient—that is, you get more energy out of carbs for a given quantity of oxygen (5.05 vs. 4.7 calories per gram for carbs and fats, respectively). Carbs are like using a higher-octane fuel, resulting in more bang for the buck. If you want to exercise intensely and you eat a low-carb diet, you will not be able to perform at your highest level. If you're eating enough calories to cover your body's basal needs and your exercise use, you can get by with 40 percent or less of your calories coming from carbs. Eating more than that will not necessarily benefit exercise (it's not a case of some is good, so more is better). I do believe that most people who are training overdo the carbs, however, given the limited amount and intensity of training that they do. It's an undeniable fact that it takes 24–48 hours to fully restore muscle glycogen if you deplete any during exercise, and that time frame assumes that you're eating adequate amounts of carbs. If you're on a low-carb dietary regimen, it will inevitably take longer, and you may be trying to do your next work- out with less muscle and liver glycogen available. Being glycogen depleted also does not necessarily improve your fat use because, as we say in the exer- cise physiology world, "fat burns in a carbohydrate flame." If your muscles are glycogen depleted, your fat use will be somewhat compromised, and you'll have to slow down your pace for that reason as well.

Low-carb eating and exercise has not been well studied in diabetic individuals, but let me give you a recent published example of its effects in a non-diabetic popu- lation during a single session of exercise to exhaustion done at a high intensity. Keep in mind that this study is related to optimal performance at a higher level, not the mild or moderate activity done during an average exercise session like brisk walking for an hour. The study, published in Brazilian Journal of Medical and Biological Research *in late 2009, examined the effects of lowering carbohydrate intake for 48 hours and its effect on the time to exhaustion during moderate and heavy exercise. Seven men participated in a randomized order in two diet and exercise regimens, each lasting three days with a one-week interval for washout. After doing a glycogen-depleting bout of exercise, the men ate a diet with either 10 percent or 65 percent of calories derived from carbohydrates for the two days before testing. The researchers found that subjects only had problems with early fatigue during the higher-intensity exercise done in a more glycogen-depleted state, but not during the lower-intensity exercise. They concluded that this finding may be related to an inability of fat oxidation to substitute for muscle glycogen oxidation at high exercise intensities. The glycogen-depleted subjects did have a greater fat use during exercise, but the exercise also felt harder to them (i.e., their perceived effort with low glycogen levels was higher).*

Admittedly, if all of your exercise training and competing is going to be done at a submaximal level (with your goal being just to finish and not to be competitive), then this study may not be that relevant to you. Do you really need to restrict carbs so severely if you're exercising regularly? Probably not. Even people with type 2 diabetes will be able to handle some carbs better when doing regular physical activity that depletes some muscle glycogen (the main storage depot for excess carbohydrate consumption), and they may feel less tired and more energetic when eating some carbs during and/or after exercise in particular to speed up muscle glycogen repletion. On rest days, a lower carb diet is certainly better for everyone (even people without diabetes). For individuals with type 1 diabetes, it's also critical to keep your blood sugars in good control to optimize muscle and liver glycogen restoration; it won't be effectively restored if your sugars are running too high. Taking in some carbs post-exercise is probably the most important time—during that "window of opportunity" from thirty minutes to two hours afterwards when glycogen repletion rates are highest—which is also when you'll need the least amount of insulin to cover any carbs you eat. It doesn't necessarily have to be a lot; you can start out with maybe 15 to 30 grams, depending on how long and hard you worked out. I have to reiterate, though, that your body cannot process fat as quickly or as efficiently as carbs during exercise (the lower number of calories derived from oxygen per gram of fat is a non-disputable fact), so you will never reach your peak performance for high-intensity exercise relying on fats alone. If you can still do less intense exercise as well as you'd like to while using more fats than carbs and optimal performance is not your concern, then a low-carb lifestyle and exercise may work just fine for you.

If you need tips for getting started on an exercise program, check out my book entitled The 7 Step Diabetes Fitness Plan. *For people with any type of diabetes who are already more active, you will benefit more from* Diabetic Athlete's Handbook.

I started running when I was fifteen years old, after I was diagnosed with diabetes. When I asked my doctor if that meant I couldn't play sports, I'd been hoping for an excuse to miss field hockey practice, he laughed and told me exercise would help keep my blood sugars in check. So when the field hockey season ended, I started running. As the years passed, I began to call myself "a runner."

I bought running shoes from a real running shoe store, learned how to properly stretch and cool down. I was happy to discover that running improved my blood sugars and decided it was time to enter my first race. I sent in money for a 5K and the morning of the race, as I neared the finish line, I couldn't wait to race again.

Slowly, I began collecting race tee-shirts and recognizing faces at local runs. When a fellow runner mentioned she was going to a Team in Training meeting, I decided to go along. By the next weekend, I found myself at six in the morning standing at the edge of a downtown lake with a group of strangers. Our plan was to run eight miles. I panicked as the group set off at a fast pace, worried that I was not ready. What if my blood sugar got low, what if I couldn't keep up? I didn't look like a runner; I was tall and had big feet that seemed to smack the pavement instead of springing from it like my friend who moved ambitiously to the head of the pack. By the time we reached our first water stop, I was solidly in the middle of the pack, breathing hard, my legs burning, but feeling strong.

Every week I drove to my friend's house and we ran from one end of the island and back. I carried a rolled up dollar in my shorts to buy a Gatorade in case I got low, or a small bag of Skittles that always melted by the end of the run. Every Sunday from September to December, we met our group at the lake and ran farther than the week before. During this time I followed a trial-and-error eating plan. The night before our long runs, I always carbo-loaded because that's what everyone else on my training team was doing. Only I was the only one with diabetes. I enjoyed the fact that I "had" to eat a bowl of pasta the night before the long runs because I normally avoided pasta and somehow, during all those months, it never occurred to me to eat any differently. I'm sure I woke up with higher than normal blood sugars, but I always gave myself a shot, ate my carbo-filled cereal breakfast, and headed out the door to run ten, fifteen, or twenty miles.

When the morning of the marathon finally arrived, I woke up early, tested my blood sugar and was horrified to discover that it was 250. I'd flown to Disney World the day before, and eaten a big bowl of pasta for dinner with my family. Right before bed I was low and had juice and graham crackers. I didn't want to wake up in the middle of the night needing sugar. That morning, I gave an extra big shot, ate my normal breakfast of cereal, and headed to the start line. The first two hours of the marathon were tough. I was groggy, heavy, and thirsty because of my blood sugar. By mile ten, my sugar finally felt like it was stabilizing and I began to feel a spike in energy, and then I hit the wall at mile twenty as my body quaked with fatigue and my blood sugar crashed. I picked up a bottle of Gatorade and a power bar at the next drink station and had to stop and walk. I felt terrible. I thought I'd never make it to the end and picking up my feet to run again felt momentous.

I made it to the finish line in 4 hours and 45 minutes and it was one of the hardest things I've ever done. I've learned so much since then, and now I never run without a bottle of glucose tabs. I also never eat a huge plate of pasta the night before a long run. As a forty-one-year-old old mom to three boys, I also no longer have time to run for hours on end but one day I'd like to run a half marathon again. This time I will follow Sheri's advice, and I'd like to believe my run, even though I'm older, will be that much stronger.

But what if you are not exercising? Does that mean you shouldn't eat carbs? What if you need to lose weight but have a hard time committing to an exercise program? Are carbs off limits? The debate continues.

What's with all the hype? The biggest frustration for me surrounding low carbs is the controversy. I could never understand why people get so fired up about the topic until I started to change the way I thought about food.

Michelle Sorensen says, "I think that weight is a huge issue in our society and people want to believe they can eat the foods they find satisfying and still lose weight ... for many North Americans, sadly, those foods are fatty or sugary. So people like the idea that you can cut out carbs but it is okay to eat cheeseburgers with bacon ... just drop the bun! People lose weight but are consuming diets high in animal fat, which increases the risk of heart disease and other illnesses regardless of your weight. Some people are on the other extreme, bashing low-carb diets because they are addicted to the baked goods and sweets in their diet and don't want to give them up. Sadly, not enough people learn that whole, plant-based and natural foods can be delicious and satisfying and low carb. When I fill my plate with vegetables, legumes, and sometimes some grains, I am getting what I need without worrying about how many carbohydrates I consume.

"I used to be hooked on carbohydrates and it took some really hard work to change that. When I had to eat gluten free, I started by eating healthier carbs and then gradually, as I learned how to incorporate more vegetables, beans, and lentils in my diet, I didn't need as much rice, pasta, white potato, etc. I feel much better for it."

Franziska says, "I think the reason low-carb diets are so controversial is because they're not really accepted by the ADA and the Academy of Nutrition and Dietetics, though recently the ADA endorsed them as a method for weight control if used for no more than one year. It has been said that the body requires 130 grams of carbohydrates to meet the absolute needs of the brain; however, a portion of this can be derived via gluconeogenesis, assuming protein and caloric needs are met. In my opinion, sometimes being too vocal about low carb being the only way to manage diabetes can turn people off. That being said, I do feel it's the best method for managing blood sugar levels."

Sysy says she thinks the carb controversy has more to do with a concern over high blood sugars. "Most low-carb dieters eat a lot of animal protein and fat, which has been deemed unhealthy in large quantities by the medical community. However, I believe that many people make the decision to eat that way because they feel that high blood sugars are more damaging to the body than a low-carb, high-fat and protein diet. They feel the trade off is worth it. For those who feel healthy eating this way, I imagine their health can't be too bad. When we're not healthy, our energy levels and overall feelings of wellness instinctively let us know."

Rachel says,"I think there are some definite dangers to low-carb dieting. For one, I have rarely met a person who goes on a diet and has a healthy attitude about eating and their body before, during, and afterward. Low-carb dieting involves eating a lot of protein. I've done a lot of research on foods and how they are grown or butchered or harvested, and it's pretty scary stuff. There are tons of unhealthy chemicals and hormones in our foods. Our family chooses to eat organic as much as possible. I think if someone is going to go low carb, go quality low-carb—meaning, buy organic. Yes, it's a lot more money, but pay for it now or pay for it later."

Elizabeth says she understands the hype surrounding low-carb diets. "They provide quick results if you're trying to lose weight and are typically easy to maintain if you're into eating meat all the time. They are also a good way to help your blood sugar levels to stabilize. Low carbs is less insulin, which is less room for error. The two weeks I was on the Dukan diet my Dexcom showed an essentially flat line. I was amazed. But I was hungry for a croissant."

DO FEWER CARBS EQUAL BETTER BLOOD SUGAR CONTROL?

One of the most common reasons for decreasing carbs among people living with diabetes is improved blood sugar control. The less carbs you eat, the less insulin you need.

Sysy says she definitely has better blood sugar control with a low-carb diet. "Every time we inject or bolus insulin a varying percentage of insulin is not absorbed by the body. This amount increases as the amount of insulin given increases and this means that if we eat fewer carbs and give less insulin, we have less dramatic blood sugar variation to deal with. I don't view this as opinion as much as I do fact. Obviously, there are factors that might make it hard or impossible for someone to lessen carbohydrates. But, I credit lowering carbs with my much improved blood sugar management. In fact, I didn't eat the American Diabetic Association's recommendation of carbs while pregnant with my twins and everything went well."

Rachel says, "Lower-carb eating does help me control my blood sugars and maintain my weight. My energy level is higher because I'm not yo-yoing between carbs and insulin and insulin and carbs. I wish I had the discipline to go on a lower-carb diet, but right now, I cannot fathom giving up the few things I truly enjoy—fruits and healthy desserts."

Q&A WITH FRANZISKA SPRITZLER, RD, CDE

You are a CDE and and RD and maintain the website, Low Carb Dietitian. You also work at the VA Medical Center in Los Angeles. So I would imagine that you work with a wide variety of patients. Can you tell me what you would recommend to someone who wants to get started on a lower-carb diet? I'm sure it depends on the individual and that individual's personal goals, but can you give me a general idea of how to get started?

I generally recommend cutting down on carbohydrates gradually and using a glucometer to track how different amounts of carbs affect blood sugar. It would to some extent depend on how many carbs the person is currently consuming, but overall I'd say cutting down to 40 grams per meal is a good place to start. Some may find enough improvement at this level to remain there; 120 grams per day is still considered low-carb by American Diabetes Association standards. If blood sugar control remains poor, I advise people to cut down by 5 grams per meal or sitting and continue to assess their one-to-two-hour postprandial levels, as well as how they feel overall. I've never counseled anyone who needed or wanted to go below 15 grams per meal, but I know Dr. Bernstein has had great results with only 6 grams at breakfast and 12 grams at lunch and dinner, both personally and with thousands of patients.

When people are diagnosed with diabetes, many of them feel overwhelmed with everything they need to learn and everything they need to change. As they become more

informed about their relationship with food and how foods affect their body, many people (type 1 and type 2) find success with a low-carb way of eating. What is the best way to make a low-carb diet simple for people with diabetes?

The way to simplify carb counting is to first get a guide to carbohydrate servings of foods (the American Diabetes Association has several) and familiarize yourself with the various carbohydrate counts of foods. Within a short time, selecting low-carb options will become automatic. On a carbohydrate-restricted diet, your meals should be based around meat/fish/protein/eggs and nonstarchy vegetables, which contain few carbs. Depending on one's personal carbohydrate target per meal, small amounts of fruit, dairy, and nuts are added to achieve the amount of carbs desired.

Aside from providing fuel and nourishment, eating is enjoyable, social, and comforting. A low-carb diet shouldn't be seen as a deprivation diet. Many "comfort foods" fit into a low-carb plan: sausage and eggs, peanut butter, guacamole, and steak are just a few examples. However, overeating is unhealthy, even if foods are low in carbohydrates. Striking a balance is key.

We need energy to fuel our body during exercise. I remember when I was training for my marathon in 1995 with Team in Training, it was recommended that we "carbo-load" before races. Eating a big bowl of pasta like my fellow runners never worked for me, all it did was raise and then lower my blood sugar. What do you recommend to your patients when it comes to a low-carb diet and exercise?

I recommend regular low-to-moderate-intensity exercise for 20 to 40 minutes on a daily basis. Those on insulin and oral hypoglycemic meds should test their sugar before and after exercise to prevent lows. The best time to exercise is one to two hours after eating, when blood glucose tends to be highest.

Can you tell me your thoughts on the sustainability of a low-carb diet for your patients over the long term, and how does this way of eating work for busy families? Also, is a low-carb way of eating more expensive?

I think a low-carb diet can be maintained over the long term fairly easily. Initially there will probably be an adjustment period when planning meals may seem difficult. However, soon it will become second nature. High-carbohydrate foods like rice, pasta, and potatoes can still be prepared for children or spouses of people following carb restriction. Overall, low-carbing shouldn't be more expensive than a traditional diet. Foods like canned tuna or salmon, eggs, chicken drumsticks, lean cuts of meat, peanut butter, and frozen vegetables are very reasonably priced. Purchasing meat and cheese on sale is also a great way to stretch your dollars on a low-carb plan.

Snacks are a big challenge for people wanting to follow a low-carb diet. What other than nuts do you recommend?

Some of my favorite low-carb snacks are string cheese, peanut butter on celery, olives, cottage cheese, and guacamole on slices of red bell pepper.

In his book, *The Sweet Life: Diabetes Without Borders*, Sam Talbot shares his recipe for the low-carb snack, Kale chips:

2 large bunches (about 2-½ pounds) kale, stems and center ribs discarded, leaves roughly torn
2 sheets nori, cut into 1″ × 2″ strips
¼ cup roasted garlic oil
1 teaspoon coarse sea salt
½ teaspoon freshly ground black pepper
Zest of 1 lemon

(continued)

Kale Chips (continued)

Preparation

Preheat the oven to 350°F. Line a baking sheet with tin foil or parchment paper.

In a large bowl, toss the kale and nori with the oil until coated. Then spread the kale and nori on the lined baking sheet and sprinkle with the salt and pepper. Bake for 6 to 8 minutes or until the kale and nori are crispy. Be careful not to cook much longer, or the nori and kale will turn dark and bitter.

Remove the baking sheet from the oven and sprinkle the kale and nori with the lemon zest. Let the chips cool to room temperature before serving.

Serves 4–6

When transitioning to a low-carb diet, do patients need to be aware of lows? Should they work with their doctors and/or certified diabetes educator (CDE) while making this transition? Aren't they more apt to have lows and need less insulin on a low-carb diet?

Patients should always be aware of the possibility of lows and make sure they have glucose or a form of rapid-acting carbohydrate with them at all times. I do think patients on insulin or hypoglycemic agents should work with a doctor, pharmacist, dietitian, or CDE while making the transition because dosage will in all likelihood need to be reduced. If med dosages are not changed, a person may definitely experience a low. However, if dosages are adjusted, people are less apt to have lows because fewer carbs require less insulin, which results in more predictable blood sugars.

Do you worry at all about all the good and bad eating advice that can be found online? Why are there so many different opinions when it comes to eating right and how can patients know whom to trust and where to find the "right" information?

Yes, there are all kinds of diets and eating plans found online, and some of them are unbalanced and in some cases dangerous. It's hard to know which ones to trust. In general, advice from doctors and dietitians can be relied on, although their recommendations can certainly differ. I think it's good that there are different options because we're all so unique. Carbohydrate restriction works well for me and for many others, but it's not for everyone. A diet that is balanced, satisfying, and contains both plant and animal foods, essential fats, and fiber is optimal, regardless of the amount of carbohydrate it contains.

Ann Rosenquist Fee says, "When the Atkins diet got huge, I got mad. I'd been eating that way for years—salads with no croutons, plain yogurt with stevia, Crystal Light/Jack Daniels instead of Mike's Hard Lemonade (my husband called it Crisky)—and feeling awkward about it. All of a sudden here were a bunch of women's magazines making it hot. I guess I wanted some credit.

"I didn't stay mad for long, because grocery shopping was suddenly a delight. Every aisle had something. Low-carb cookies, low-carb pancake mix. I think there were even Glycemic Index guides in the produce section (bananas, bad; apples, good). The Atkins frozen dinners were divine. They didn't taste great, but they made me feel normal. A frozen dinner. Look at me. Eating processed microwaveables just like everybody else.

"I was happy until everybody went gluten free. Then I got mad again, but this time at the gluten-free people. All that rice-based stuff, are you kidding me? Dr. Atkins, please, make a comeback. Give me high-protein lasagna in a plastic tray and make it hot."

AUTHENTIC ADVICE

■ *Diets don't work, ever, period. A lifestyle does work. And I think diabetics have to get out of the mindset of dieting and radically change their lifestyles for life.* ■ Rachel Garlinghouse

■ *What I would like people to consider is not a low-carb diet, but a nonprocessed-food diet. I've found that not eating processed food lowers carbs immensely because of how fat and fiber and the glycemic index in foods impacts our bodies. I wish there would be less wars on low-carb versus high-carb and more conversations about processed foods and whole foods and how they function in the body.* ■ Sysy Morales

5   Eating Mindfully

Even though I joke that my dad forced me into vegetarianism when I was a kid, I'm serious when I say that he showed me there is pleasure in food, even for a woman with diabetes. Being diagnosed with diabetes as a teenager, I had two strikes against me when it came to food. Strike one: As women, we are not supposed to love food. Instead, we eat salads, skip breakfast, and say no to desserts. Strike two: As diabetics, food is a science and we must count carbs, measure insulin ratios to carbohydrate intake, and use language like *food exchanges*, *sugar-free*, and *moderation* to discuss what we put in our mouths. But long before I was diagnosed, my dad laid the foundation of a love of food that has stuck with me over the years. Sometimes it was only a faint reminder, but more recently his love of food has become a powerful ray that I draw on as I continue to shape the way I think about eating well with diabetes.

My relationship with food began with my hippie parents. We lived on one hundred acres of woods in Vermont and raised chickens, pulled vegetables from the garden, and composted the remains (the browned bananas, the hardened tips of green beans, and the moldy tomatoes) that were tossed on top of the pile in the back yard. Dad said that when my sister and I were hungry, all we needed to do was go outside. Every spring, he drove me to the bottom of our dirt road to visit Hazen Clay, an ancient looking Vermont farmer, in his sugaring shack. We walked through the crusty snow across the cow field to the small, wooden shack with smoke pouring out of a chimney on the roof. In my moon boots, I could almost walk the whole way without falling through the snow. Even though it was March, it was still cold, and my breath came out in puffs. Dad opened the door, and we entered a thick wall of heat. I unzipped my parka. In the middle of the small space was a giant tub where the syrup was cooking, and I had to stand on a bench to see. Hazen stirred the syrup with a long, metal spoon and the sugar water bubbled, light brown and thick. Finally, Dad motioned me outside and Hazen passed us each a small silver bowl from his shelf. We scooped up crusty snow and Hazen poured the thick liquid over the top. The first bite was always a surprise, a strange mixture of textures and sensations—the crunchy, cold snow and the still hot, too sweet syrup. I shivered, and ate another bite.

I used to think of that maple syrup after I was diagnosed and wanted Dad's famous animal pancakes for breakfast. My sister also had type 1 diabetes and so Mom replaced Hazen's maple syrup with the sugar-free kind that tasted like water. I hated the sugar-free syrup and stopped eating pancakes. But I missed the syrup. I missed the special trips to Hazen's sugar shack that suddenly disappeared. I missed saying yes to food. Dad never stopped offering me bites, but it wasn't the same when only a bite was allowed. I was angry, and resentful, and tired of saying no.

It's been twenty-six years since I was diagnosed, and only recently that I have begun saying yes to food again. Yes to raw green beans from the farmer's market, yes to bell peppers, plums, cherries, cheese, avocado, turkey bacon, peanuts, and dark chocolate. Now that I am a mother, I want to reach out my hand holding a spoon and offer my children a bite. I want to watch my sons Will, Miles, and Reid close their eyes in pleasure, whether it's over the peanut butter we've ground in the machine at the local health food store, or the strawberries we've picked off the vine or even the candy that they love: Air Heads, Candy Corn, Pez, and Reese's Peanut Butter Cups. I want to teach them a love of food like my dad taught me, whether I take a bite or not, because if we love what we eat, according to expert Megrette Fletcher, we will treat it with respect and have enough, not too much, so we feel good when we're done. Like the children's book, *A Fish Out of Water* by Helen Palmer (based on a short story by Palmer's husband the famous Dr. Seuss) that teaches a lesson of balance. It's one of my boys' favorite books that teaches kids about feeding their fish the right amount: "never feed him a lot, so much and no more, or something may happen, you never know what" the book warns. Of course the boy feeds the fish too much and it grows so big that the fire department has to transport the fish to a local pool. The book is a great lesson for all things in life, take what you need, not more, or chaos ensues.

"Mindful Eating," the latest "it-girl" phrase in the nutrition world, offers a similar message as the *Fish Out of Water* book. It has its roots in Eastern philosophy and involves a greater awareness of food. In *Eat What You Love, Love What You Eat with Diabetes*, co-author Megrette Fletcher, MEd, RD, CDE, says mindful eating means something different for everyone. "Mindful Eating is eating with intention *and* attention. Intention is to address hunger and cravings, and attention is being aware of how food tastes, and our change (or approach) to hunger and fullness."

But how do we eat mindfully when we have diabetes? How do we address our hunger and cravings when our blood sugar is high or low? After years of counting carbs, how do we think abut food as something other than medicine? After years of saying no, how do we say yes to food?

Megrette Fletcher, MEd, CDE, RD, began thinking about Mindful Eating when she started meditating on a daily basis in 1999. That prompted her to write her first book, called *Discover Mindful Eating*, which was geared toward professionals. "I realized as I spent more time exploring mindfulness we needed a large nonprofit to get back to enjoying food. In 2005, I reached out to experts throughout the United States to form a nonprofit, which is TCME, based in New Hampshire. That's how I met Michelle May, a family doctor and co-author of *Eat What You Love, Love What You Eat.*"

Megrette saw *Eat What You Love, Love What You Eat* and said, "We need this book for people with diabetes." Michelle asked why, and Megrette said, "Because all your yo-yo dieters grow up to be people with diabetes. When we don't resolve our issues with food and eating, we wind up not having a good relationship with food, and end up using food when we're not hungry, and over time, oftentimes, we find ourselves with diabetes." Working together on the new book, *Eat What You Love, Love What You Eat with Diabetes*, helped Megrette realize how much guilt and shame and anger and short sightedness we have around food and eating. "It's very short sighted to feel guilty for enjoying dessert. That isn't what it's about; it's about living your life to the fullest. So the hope with this book is that it will help people have the food that they eat fuel their life, and not fuel guilt and regret." This doesn't mean eliminating carbs or only eating salad: this means learning to love food again. "If I can bring that love and passion back to people with diabetes, it would be an honor." Restricting food is never going to be the solution, we need to love food more because things you love, you value. "I love food! I love eating!" Megrette laughs.

Catherine Vancak agrees and says, "Taste is a huge part of why I choose a food! If it doesn't taste good then why would I waste the calories? With diabetes, food can certainly seem like medicine, as it is what saves us after low blood sugars. What works for me is actually designating a specific food for the treatment of low blood sugars and label that as medicine and leaving the rest of the food in my pantry as normal food. I never treat lows with my real food, I only treat [with] glucose tabs and a specific protein bar. By doing this I think it takes the pressure off of the real food. Real food doesn't need to treat my low blood sugars and instead is my fuel for the day and enjoyment."

Asha Brown founder of the We Are Diabetes website, was diagnosed with type 1 diabetes when she was five years old. She says, "I categorize my food into two different zones in regard to my diabetes: The 'medicine' I need to treat a low, and the food I use to nourish myself during a meal. When I'm low I treat it with juice, glucose tabs, and maybe some dried or fresh fruit if I need it. Then I stop. I don't turn it into a meal. I give myself time to let my body and my mind catch up so that when I do decide what to eat for a meal I can reconnect to the person, the girl, the actress, the yogi, the friend, the wife, and see what I am craving. I am not just my diabetes. I have a personality that reaches farther and deeper than fat grams and carb counts and when I allow the other facets of my life to surface in making decisions for what I want to eat, I don't feel guilt or shame for wanting what I want. I find that when I eat what I truly want, I eat as much as my body needs. This allows me to have physical and emotional balance. My weight and body image has never been better since I embraced the practice of mindful eating."

Q & A WITH MEGRETTE FLETCHER

You say mindful eating is partly about making people aware of hunger, what about people with diabetes whose hunger signals are often a sign not of hunger but of a low or high blood sugar? How can we help people to be mindful of their body's signals when those signals often don't have anything to do with hunger. Also, people with diabetes can have less effective amylin production, which influences feelings of hunger. How can we tackle these mixed and often frustrating signals?

There were a few studies published that looked at hunger, Campinalli showed that training people with diabetes to recognize and respond to initial hunger improved blood sugar control. Additionally, weight loss was noted.

It is important to note that mindful eating is greater than hunger and fullness training. These are internal cues. Mindful eating is awareness of information that is both internal and externally generated. Learning to listen and process this information without judgment (i.e., your hunger is not bad—it is just information; your blood sugar is not bad, it is just information) is really the goal! See all as information, including the internal cues, which are often not discussed in a typical diabetes appointment.

Mindful eating also stresses taste and being grateful and thinking about food as a source of nourishment. Again, how can we apply this way of thinking to diabetes where food is often seen as medicine?

Again, realizing that people all over the world suffer from diabetes, imagine how hard it would be to have diabetes if you lived in a place where there was war or limited electricity? How about if there was a food shortage like in India? You see, living in the United States is a great blessing. You and I both remember what it was like to have diabetes before meters, before pens, before pumps. Diabetes is difficult but there have been HUGE improvements in both the technology and the food labeling. Counting carbohydrates may take time, but at least we know what causes blood sugar to rise. And now foods have labels! There really is so much to be grateful for! If people realized that it was a lot harder to have diabetes in 1930, '50, '70, '90 … it can be very helpful to tolerate the day-to-day grind of diabetes now. If we add to this awareness the understanding that YOU DON'T HAVE TO EAT FOODS THAT TASTE BAD for your diet—WOW! That is huge. Back then, there really wasn't a choice. We have so much choice now!

Weight loss is a primary focus for many people with type 2 diabetes. In your blog you said: *The goal of diabetes self-management is to manage your blood sugars to allow you to live a full and vibrant life. To achieve this goal, I encourage my clients to stop focusing on an outcome and start focusing on behaviors.* **Can you explain this to me? What kind of behaviors do you recommend to clients?**

Behaviors are what you are doing NOW. Outcomes are what people did. They cannot be changed. So—what are you doing? Are you checking in with your hunger before you eat, while eating? Give it a try and see if you change what you eat. Are you thinking about how you can move your body more … what would feel good? Are you checking your blood sugar. A1Cs give an average. Your blood sugar, and getting into the idea of being CURIOUS about the number and not JUDGING it, is a behavior.

Low-carb eating gets a lot of attention in the diabetes world, yet on your blog you recommend: 45 to 75 grams of carbs eaten three times a day. As someone who has learned about eating carbs through trial and error, 75 per meal seems like a lot. Can you explain to me your philosophy on eating carbs?

Many people choose to eat less carbs because they have learned that it doesn't work for them. GREAT! I am 100 percent cool with this decision. However, there is no reason to be afraid of carbs. Especially whole grain, nutrient-rich carbs like beans and dairy and whole grains.

People with diabetes often get stuck in the blame game. I like what you say here: *It is important to see your glucose test results as clues that help you solve the mystery of how eating affects your diabetes. Resist blame, guilt, and restriction. Instead, explore possible connections between what you ate and what happens to your blood sugar.* **This is, of course, easier said that done. Can you offer some suggestions on how people with diabetes can change the negative way of thinking about blood sugar numbers?**

Practice the behavior of forgiveness. Everyone is human. We can't change that. Acknowledge that perfection is NOT how to live a vibrant life. It is how you will become crazy, angry, and depressed.

What are some of the most important steps people with diabetes can take to move away from unhealthy eating habits toward a mindful way of eating?

Pause before you eat. Ask, *am I hungry?* Take a deep breath whenever you can. Forgive yourself if you are tempted to blame yourself for something. DON'T MISS THE LESSON! Regarding high or low blood sugars—Thomas Edison said,"I didn't fail 1,999 times before I invented the light bulb, I just learned 1,999 times how NOT to build a light bulb!" See, it is all in how you look at it. Keep at it! Return to the practice of being present!

According to Megrette, mindful eating means choosing to become aware and using that info to guide food choices in a way that feels healthy. She uses eating chocolate chip cookies as an example. "What is my experience when I mindlessly snack on raw cookie dough when I'm cooking? I love cookies, but how can I eat them in a way that I feel good? I want to love them when I'm done eating them. When can I eat cookies when I won't be sacrificing my health? … when I'm low or before I exercise. Identify where you can incorporate cookies so you don't feel like your health is being sacrificed. These are the questions we have to ask over and over again. When we're feeling deprived we have more cravings then when we're not feeling deprived.

"Research out of Italy shows that overweight subjects who were trained to have an awareness of hunger and blood glucose showed long-term weight loss. The findings of this study suggest that the current epidemic of insulin resistance and obesity may have its origin in the 'non-cognizance of hunger.' By restoring and validating hunger awareness, the IHMP (initial hunger meal pattern) could help in the prevention and treatment of diabetes and obesity and a range of associated disorders, and thus lessen the high economic burden of health services in industrialized societies."

Megrette says hunger changes with each bite you take. "I describe it like a road. You start at one place and with each mile you are closer to your destination. If we use this analogy on food, knowing where you are going, your intended destination of comfortable fullness, and being aware on the way, paying attention to taste, texture, and enjoyment during the journey, you will more likely wind up at comfortable, healthy fullness. The best part is that bringing intention/attention transforms the journey from a chore into an exciting, fun, joyful part of life. What could be better?"

Asha Brown is proof that eating with intention is important for women with diabetes and says, "When I'm having a low blood sugar and I start to treat it, I do feel like I could eat everything and anything in sight. When I choose to be mindful of the fact that it doesn't take that much to treat a low, even if the emotional part of me says I need more, I find that it's easier to get a piece of fruit or juice, to let it work and get AWAY from the kitchen and the temptation to eat more. After 15 or 20 minutes I'll test again and then if I'm still hungry make a choice to eat more. If I eat more than I need when I'm low, I am not honoring my body or my diabetes because my blood sugar will spike, which can also create false hunger signals for diabetics, and I will have roller-coaster blood sugars for the rest of the day. If I'm going to eat, I want to enjoy it and not have to gulp it down because I am having a low. If I'm going to eat and take insulin and go through the effort of figuring out how much insulin I need to cover what I'm eating, then I feel like I should make every effort to have the time to enjoy that process after my low has been treated and I am thinking clearly."

Catherine Vancak was diagnosed with type 1 diabetes in 2011, just as her ballet career was taking off. She says mindful eating has been helpful to her because when you have diabetes it's not only about paying attention to your body's hunger or satiety, but also paying attention to your blood sugar while eating. "I use the number my meter gives me as a window into my body. By knowing exactly what that number is I can then ask myself, *am I really hungry or is my blood sugar too high or low?* It can be very difficult to know if my stomach is hungry or my blood sugar is. Some days are easier than others.

"With keeping myself mindful about what I eat, I can make it more logical, almost like a science experiment. I look at the numbers I'm given by my meter and also take into account how I am feeling. I like to figure out patterns that I fall into and perhaps may not be as healthy, so I can change them. Mindful eating has certainly tuned me into my body's signals and prevented many unhealthy choices from being made. All of this requires a great deal of mental effort but, like with any skill, with practice it becomes natural."

Asha Brown says throughout her childhood, diabetes was simply a way of life because her father had type 1 for most of his life as well. She writes that she didn't mind being a little different than her friends and never had a problem explaining her diabetes to anyone who had questions. In fact, diabetes never created an obstacle in her life until she was old enough to understand that her weight and body size were not completely under her own control. As a dancer, actress, and a fitness instructor by the time she was seventeen, Asha lived for movement and her body's ability to feel good in its own skin. After reading many articles and books that gave a daunting account of weight gain associated with insulin resistance and diabetes, Asha felt the first stirring of resentment toward a disease she felt was dooming her to an inability to have the physical strength and shape that she knew she deserved and could achieve. She started to omit insulin occasionally when it was "necessary" to get things done.

Asha now says mindful eating has helped her recover from years of disordered eating. "Mindful eating was key to recovering a healthy relationship with food for me. Living with diabetes means that food is part of your life and that can really affect some of us in a negative way. I found that when I overanalyzed every carbohydrate, every fat gram, every important nutrient that was good for diabetics and would ensure better blood sugars, I became very overwhelmed and it would lead to fast diabetes burnout. At that point I ate out of rebellion and would be drawn to all the 'off limits' foods I'd been told by doctors and the media that I shouldn't eat. After this I would feel so guilty, like I wasn't strong enough to do the right things for my diabetes. However, expecting myself to never enjoy something I was craving or to categorize food based on 'good' and 'bad' only created more of a divide between myself and food.

"During this part of my life I didn't know what really tasted good, what my body craved, I only knew what I should be eating, so I forced myself to think that's what I wanted to eat. Now that I let my body's natural hunger signals and my personality help me to discover what I want to eat I feel so free. It's ironic that my freedom from an eating disorder truly healed once I just ate what made my body 'hum,' versus what was deemed acceptable by the diabetes cookbooks and the media."

Catherine agrees and says mindful eating has helped her change her relationship with food. She says, "As a professional dancer I unfortunately haven't had the most happy relationship with food. It's just part of the profession to keep your weight low. That meant counting every calorie and seeing food as this enemy crouched in attack position ready to take away your job at a moment's notice.

"Over the years I have found that by writing down the food I ate and making the conscious decision to eat or not to eat softened my relationship with food. I put myself in the driver's seat and made myself accountable for the fuel I put in my body. I am the one in control of what I feel I need. By being mindful I am better able to make healthy choices and enjoy the food I have in front of me. I see food now as the energy for me to push through rehearsals, workouts, exams, and my daily life."

Q&A WITH HEATHER NIELSEN, MA

Heather Nielsen, MA, Diabetes Coach and Counselor at Integrated Diabetes Care, LLC, and type 1 diabetic, attended the Diabetes Sisters Conference in San Diego last year and participated in a mindful eating exercise.

Can you describe the workshop for me?

Dr. Liana Abascal, clinical psychologist at the Behavioral Diabetes Institute, led us through a mindful eating exercise. It was a variation on the "raisin meditation" first popularized by Jon Kabat-Zinn through his MBSR (mindfulness-based stress reduction) course. In the exercise, we are asked to take a small bite of food. We are asked to employ all our senses to notice—mindfully!—this food item. Really look at it with beginner's mind, as though we don't know what it is and have never seen it before. Technically, we never have seen THAT raisin or M&M before! Then, we smell it, "listen" to it, roll it around in our hand/fingers, and finally, put it in the mouth. We are encouraged to let it sit in our mouths, moving it around with our tongue, noticing texture, taste, etc., before biting slowly into it, and continuing to observe what happens at each moment.

Personally, I learned this activity over ten years ago and found it powerfully, amazingly helpful! It showed me how unconscious I generally am with food. Over the duration of my MBSR class, we engaged in mindful eating a lunch together, and that was even MORE powerful, as I realized how diabetes had taken me away from the appreciation of food as food, and led me to see food as "carbs" or "calories."

As a woman with diabetes, do you think mindful eating will help with diabetes management, and if so, how are you incorporating it into your life as a busy mom?

I KNOW mindful eating helps me with my diabetes management—not that I use it all the time! But having that practice has helped me notice how and when I am eating emotionally versus for physical need. It also helps me have more joy with my food, noticing both the moment of how it tastes, and further developing the practice, helping me notice how I feel after eating certain foods. So rather than my food rules being externally driven, which can lead to resistance/rebellion/burnout/anger, my rules are much more flexibly and internally driven by what is good for me holistically. Incorporating it as a busy mom isn't so hard, as I share some mindful eating practices with my children. Don't get me wrong—my kids eat Pirate's Booty and hot dogs, too! But I've seen far too many people with disordered eating to think that my children are immune. Any boost I can give them is worth the conversation and consciousness to me.

You've interviewed mindful eating experts on your show *Transforming Diabetes*, **can you tell me what was your "take-away" message? What stuck with you, what message would you hope your listeners got from your interview?**

It's been a pleasure to meet experts in this field. From Juleeanna, an RD and dialectical-behavioral therapist, the simplest and most helpful tip was packing my snacks! Being mindful of planning for my day's needs has been REALLY helpful. Not a new reminder, of course, but one that I needed to hear when I heard it, and one that has helped me take my own food needs into consideration as I pack my daughters' lunches in the morning. I also loved Donald Altman's personal story of being in a monastery and being tempted by the chocolate bar. I think that was a lesson to me that this is not something to "master" or be "bad at." It is, like all mindful practices, something available to us at any moment. This breath. And this one. All breaths, and all bites, can be mindful.

I would NEVER push mindful eating on someone. But I DO use it in my counseling and coaching practice, and many people respond to it. Some don't want to pay that much attention. I think teaching it to children is the key to transforming our relationship with food before we build too much resistance.

As women with diabetes we train ourselves to listen and respond to external cues instead of *I'm hungry, what can I eat?* I also think food becomes about control—what I can and "can't" eat. Susan Weiner says it really helps to keep a food record. A lot of people prefer to use "apps," but I like using pen and paper. Use a small notebook that you can carry with you and won't find cumbersome. Make note of the food you eat and the time you eat it. I find it very helpful to "rate your hunger" before you eat, on a scale from 1 to 10. One being not hungry and 10 being starving. When the food journal is reviewed with an RD or CDE, emotional eating patterns can be identified. Keep a column for comments. Comments can be very helpful for understanding why we eat.

AUTHENTIC ADVICE

■ *Food is not a reward. Food is not a punishment. I discuss enjoying food with my patients, but not using it to solve emotional issues. We work on eating until satisfied, not full. This often takes practice. We work on eating sitting down, not over the sink or in front of the refrigerator. Being mindful, not neurotic.* ■ Susan Weiner

■ *It's all about you! Remember at the end of the day you are eating for your body, not someone else's. Eat food that you personally enjoy and that will keep your body running. Begin with small changes such as opening up the cupboard and asking yourself how hungry you are and what your blood sugar is. If you happen to have a low blood sugar then treat with your "medicine" and come back later if you are truly hungry.* ■ Catherine Vancak

■ *Listen to what your body truly "hums" for. What do you think would happen if you decided to have it? Take some time to notice what happens when you eat meals you think you should be eating vesus what you really want to be eating. Even if your belly is full, are you still craving what you really wanted? Also, to clarify, when I say "really want to be eating," I'm not referring to the many media-laden images of burgers, fries, junk food snacks, and desserts. I'm referring to the foods that make you FEEL good, both during the meal and after. Personally I was surprised by the discoveries I made.* ■ Asha Brown

6 Going Meatless? Is the Vegan/Vegetarian Diet Right for You?

After struggling with disordered eating behaviors throughout high school, I resolved to eat better in college and returned to a vegetarian diet. However, because of both a tight budget and lack of cooking and nutrition skills, this meant subsisting on bagels, pizza, and cheesy pasta, which was not good for my weight or my blood sugar. This was before the results of the Diabetes Control and Complications Trial were released and showed tight blood sugars would decrease diabetes-related complications. No one was pushing me to have tighter blood sugar control. Of course, as a college student I wouldn't have listened anyway; I was more interested in dollar beers on Thursday nights. I'm glad those days are over.

Now, as a forty-one-year-old mother of three, I eat a well balanced diet that includes protein, vegetables, dairy, and some fruit. I enjoy eating a variety of protein, mostly in the form of chicken, tuna, turkey, and eggs, and find that these foods do a great job of satisfying my hunger without raising my blood sugars. Sometimes, the perfect snack is a roll of deli meat. However, many of my friends are vegans, and in my ongoing struggle for good blood sugar management, I am often curious about various ways of eating right.

The benefits of a plant-based diet include:

- *Weight loss*: Vegetarian diets are often lower in calories and have fewer saturated fats. A healthy body weight can improve blood sugar control and reduce your risk of diabetes complications.
- *Improved blood sugar management*: A diet based on fruits, whole grains, legumes, and nuts can improve blood sugar control

115

and insulin sensitivity. This may result in needing less medication and a decreased risk of diabetes-related complications.

■ *Reduced risk of cardiovascular disease*: A strict vegan diet is cholesterol free, low in saturated fat, and usually high in soluble fiber. A low-fat vegetarian diet can reduce your risk of cardiovascular disease, a common complication for people with diabetes.

Michelle Sorensen was diagnosed with type 1 diabetes a few weeks before her twenty-fifth birthday. From the time she was diagnosed, she'd also suffered from gastrointestinal symptoms. After several frustrating years of trying to find a diet that would work, Michelle turned to "eating green." "When I cut out gluten, dairy, eggs, yeast, and some other foods from my diet, my goal was to heal my digestive system and relieve symptoms. I was thinking more about eliminating the culprits causing my reflux, heartburn, and other gastrointestinal symptoms. These symptoms did improve,

Michelle's Diet Consists of the Following:

■ *Breakfast*: "A green smoothie. It usually has a scoop of vegan protein powder, spinach or Swiss chard, pineapple, banana, and a bit of agave nectar to sweeten it. I also like to use frozen blueberries for a really cold smoothie."

■ *Lunch/dinner*: Michelle says lunch is usually leftovers from dinner. "We have homemade bean salad, quinoa salad, chickpea patties, vegetable curries, lentil or vegetable soups, sweet potato fries, grilled vegetables or steamed vegetables. Many of these dishes are served with basmati rice."

■ *Snacks*: "Fruit or gluten-free chips (for example, root vegetable chips). In the evening I am hungry (especially these days because I am breastfeeding twin newborns!) so I make almond milk shakes with banana and nut butter, with a little pure maple syrup for flavor. I also make homemade, gluten-free, vegan cookies."

but in addition, my energy began to improve. Over time, I started to understand that food was my medicine and could heal me. It took time to develop the insight that I needed to add in better foods in order to heal my body, not just take out the *bad* foods."

Michelle saw benefits to her digestive system with a gluten-free diet, but the changes to her blood glucose (BG) control have been greater since she evolved into a more plant-based diet with fewer fast-acting carbohydrates. "I eat less white potatoes, white rice, rice pasta, and so on. Now my plate is full of vegetables, sometimes with a smaller portion of a starchy food. My insulin needs are lower, and so I find the margin for error is less. I used to have greater lows and greater highs but now my range is better. I think a low glycemic diet is really helpful and vegetables are definitely low on the glycemic index."

A mother to four young children, Michelle says eating thoughtfully does not stop at her own plate. "I have definitely encountered some raised eyebrows and comments about 'depriving' my kids of candy, ice cream, and other goodies. They have cake at birthdays, but I just don't make a habit of having sugary foods or packaged stuff around the house. I think it is hard for people to understand unless they have suffered a health crisis like I did and had such a long journey to feeling well again, that I would do anything to protect my kids from what I endure with diabetes every day.

"When we are mindful and find joy in healthy food, we feel more alive and vibrant, we have more energy to deal with difficulties we encounter, our mood is better, and we are proud of our choices. We begin to make other good decisions. I can honestly say that besides the children I brought into this world, there is nothing I feel more pride in than the way I healed myself from an onslaught of autoimmune issues (thyroid, then diabetes, then celiac) by simply feeding myself wonderful food."

I'm not quite ready to say goodbye to my deli meats or burgers, but I am curious, and the results are persuasive.

Type 2 diabetics also benefit from a plant-based diet. Studies have shown that a low fat vegan diet improves blood sugar control and cardiovascular risks in people with type 2 diabetes. Dr. Neal Barnard, with the Department of Medicine, George Washington University, Washington, DC, and founder and president of the Physicians Committee for Responsible Medicine, Washington, DC, has studied the effects of a low-fat, vegan diet on this group. Prior studies have shown that near-vegetarian diets reduce the need for insulin and oral medications in individuals with type 2 diabetes. A low-fat, vegan diet was associated with improved glycemic control, weight loss, and improved plasma lipid control during a twenty-two-week study period.

Barnard's studies show that what is particularly critical in diabetes management is long-term improvement in clinical measures, particularly glycemia and cardiovascular risk factors. Well-planned low-fat vegan diets are nutritionally adequate and, in research studies, have shown acceptability comparable with that of other therapeutic diets, suggesting they are suitable for long-term use. In a 2008 paper about a low-fat vegan diet compared to a conventional diet Barnard's research team writes: *"The most urgent clinical question regarding therapeutic diets is not whether they work, but whether they are sustainable."*

Nutrition therapy is an essential component to diabetes management, and that's why this study sought to determine the long-term sustainability of a vegan diet and answer the questions: Can you eat this way for the long haul? It turns out that yes, participants did eat this way and did show successful blood sugar control during the seventy-four-week trial.

> *Compared with the ADA (American Dietary Association) guidelines diet, the vegan diet required slightly more initial effort, but was less likely to be described as constraining. These findings suggest that both a vegan diet and a diet following 2003 ADA guidelines meet a reasonable level of acceptability, at least among motivated individuals, although the vegan diet appears to elicit much more pronounced long-term nutritional changes.*

The study seemed to stress a change in attitude toward the vegetarian diet. "The findings of our study and previous investigations show that vegetarian and low-fat vegan diets should not be described as extreme, difficult, or unacceptable, at least among research volunteers." Barnard adds, "The ADA now accepts our method, which is also encouraging."

Tracey Starkovich Moes is vegan and says the pros are many. "I ingest no cholesterol, I save animals and the environment, and overall I'd say my health has received the benefits. Also, it forces me to make healthier food choices, not because I 'can't' eat something, but because I won't. The only con I see is that it can be hard to eat out in really mainstream places, even finding a salad I will eat is hard sometimes, but it's totally worth it."

Tracey has been experimenting with raw foods after a raw cleanse in January. "Since then I have been eating raw until dinner Monday to Friday, which equals half my total meals. As far as carbs go, I did eat more carbs for a while as I adjusted. I was a pretty carb-happy vegetarian for twelve years before going vegan. The raw meals have made it easier to back off the carbs quite a bit, as does the fact that I love all veggies. I make sure at least half my plate is veggies, and usually 1/4 carbs and 1/4 protein."

US NEWS & WORLD REPORT CHOSE THE VEGAN DIET AS THE FIFTH BEST DIET FOR PEOPLE WITH DIABETES:

- The aim: Depends, but may include weight loss, heart health, and diabetes prevention or control.
- The claim: Going vegan could help shed pounds and fend off chronic diseases.
- The theory: You can cook up a perfectly healthy, meat- and dairy-free menu that supports weight loss and reduces the risk of heart disease, diabetes, and cancer.

HOW DOES THE VEGAN DIET WORK?

While vegetarians eliminate meat, fish, and poultry, vegans take it a step further, excluding all animal products—even dairy and eggs. Vegans are often animal rights activists who don't believe in using animal products for any purpose. So say goodbye to refried beans with lard, margarine made with whey, and anything with gelatin, which comes from animal bones and hooves, too. Fruits, vegetables, leafy greens, whole grains, nuts, seeds, and legumes will be your staples.

WHAT YOU'LL EAT

Going vegan means dropping all animal products—meat, fish, even dairy. It's up to you to shape a nutritionally sound diet based on fruits, veggies, leafy greens, whole grains, nuts, seeds, and legumes. Each day, you'll aim for six servings of grains; five servings of legumes, nuts, and other types of protein, like tofu; four servings of veggies; two servings of fruit; and two servings of healthy fats. With some creativity and work, you can find ways to continue eating your favorites. Try vegan cupcakes made without butter, eggs, and albumin, for example. Though restaurant meals are possible, dining out is a challenge, so prepare for lots of time in the kitchen.

In her article for *Diabetes Health*, "Veganism and Diabetes," Lisa Robertson writes,

> *As I was sitting in the hospital after a heart attack, my cardiologist walked in and said, "You have to stop eating meat."*
>
> *"Red meat?" I asked hopefully.*
>
> *"All meat," he replied firmly. It was disconcerting, to say the least, because meat has been in my life since I could feed myself. But my cardiologist explained, "If you don't want to end up back here again, you will start on a plant-based diet immediately." That day,*

I stopped eating meat. In fact, I asked the hospital food service to switch me to a vegetarian diet.

At the time, I didn't understand the overwhelming emotional and physical impact this change would have on my life and family. Until something is gone, you don't know how much you will miss it. The experience has been like a bad break-up: You miss it, you want it back, and everything reminds you that it's gone. But one thing I can say is that my health has improved. It has been only three months, but I can already see a difference in myself, my husband, and my children. My decision to change my lifestyle has impacted not only my everyday life, but also my life with diabetes. I have had diabetes for over 10 years, and the hardest part is still the fluctuation in my sugar levels on a day-to-day basis. Changing from a complete carnivore to a vegan has had a major impact on my sugar levels, which go down quickly on some days but not on other days. Planning meals has become a big part of my life, and it still takes up a lot of my time. Over the last three months, I have struggled with designing meals that will help both my diabetes and my heart disease.

If you are planning on making the change to veganism, prepare yourself for the ups and downs that will follow. Easing into it will make the change less emotionally and physically overwhelming.

THE FOLLOWING TIPS MAY PROVE HELPFUL IF YOU ARE PLANNING TO BECOME A VEGAN:

- Check your blood sugar regularly.
- Check the amount of sugar and carbs in the fruits and vegetables that you eat.

(continued)

THE FOLLOWING TIPS MAY PROVE HELPFUL IF YOU ARE PLANNING TO BECOME A VEGAN: (continued)

- Eat six small meals instead of three larger ones.
- If you are exercising more, check your sugar levels before, during, and after each workout.
- Drink plenty of water.
- Carry a snack with you at all times.
- Reduce your juice intake if you increase your fruit intake.
- Most important of all, don't worry if you slip up. Becoming vegan is a total life change, and we all know that change doesn't happen overnight!

When you reduce your meat and carbohydrate intake, you tend to overdo the fruits and vegetables to feel full. But when you have diabetes, you must watch the natural sugars in foods as well. Checking your blood sugar more frequently will ensure that your sugar levels are not going too low or high.

As my cardiologist explained, "Meat creates additional plaque in the arteries, causing a narrowing of the arteries and blood vessels that can lead to heart attack and stroke. A vegan diet reduces the chances of future plaque build-up. While being a vegan can't undo the damage that is already done, I believe that it can prevent further damage from occurring. I don't know if the plaque is clearing from my arteries yet. But I do know that I feel far better now than I have in a long time. Making the switch to veganism has been a hard road, but the payoff is well worth it."

In an interview with Jessica Apple, co-founder of *A Sweet Life*, Adrian Kiger, who was diagnosed with type 1 diabetes when she was eleven years old, talks about her switch to a plant-based diet. Included here is an excerpt from their conversation.

Adrian says, "A few years ago, I started dating a strict vegan who had been committed to his lifestyle for twenty years when I met him. I was intrigued by his dedication to it. I was also open to trying something new at the time. I knew that my health had been in a holding-pattern: I was managing, but not thriving with diabetes.

"I was confident that trying veganism would help me focus in on a very specific way of eating which would serve me and my diabetes. I also knew that the numerous chunks of cheese in my fridge weren't doing my waistline any favors and that cheese and crackers were a convenient comfort food for me. Beyond that, I could do without eggs, and was already drinking soy milk. (I've since switched to unsweetened almond milk, which has a minimal impact on my sugar levels.)

"Going vegan meant the simplification of food choices. I didn't feel so overwhelmed at grocery stores, because I knew what sections to totally avoid. You really hone in on the healthiest stuff as a vegan shopper: fruits and veggies, beans and grains, nuts and seeds. These foods give your body so many nutrients."

Adrian says her A1C has improved and now stays put at 7 or below. "This also has to do with steering clear of carbohydrates that cause spikes, and eating the more natural ones. I also think that a hemoglobin A1C reading is not the holy grail of your overall sugar control; it is an average. I used to eat a lot more food that was not as healthy as what I eat now, and my A1C would still show up normal, because it was an average of highs and a lot of lows."

Adrian doesn't see following a vegan diet and living with diabetes as *restrictive*.

"I felt from the very beginning that living with diabetes and being vegan is a sort of double whammy. Diabetes is hard enough. I didn't think of it so much as denying myself, because you can make any dish vegan, but those dishes are not often easily accessible, you have to make them yourself. This means more work, more thought in your preparation. However, as diabetics, we already have to plan ahead, so planning to eat vegan food just becomes part of that. But when you're tired and hungry, or you're at a work event and the carrot sticks aren't enough for you, and what's in the salad dressing is a mystery ... well then, I break down and eat something with dairy in it. Because of this, I don't advertise that I am a 'vegan,' because I am not a strict vegan. I accept that there will always be that moment that I fall off of the wagon, so to speak. My priority is balancing my blood sugar with living and enjoying my life to the fullest. I roll with how my body feels, give it what it needs. And I recognize that what it needs and wants are two different things entirely."

Wants and needs are very different things, like Adrian says, and it's up to us as individuals to determine what our body needs.

Rachel Garlinghouse was a vegetarian in high school, and then she started eating meat again because her diet lacked protein. "My doctor, at the time, saw how horribly my blood sugars were swinging (this was pre-diabetes) and told me that not eating meat was contributing to the problem. However, two years ago, I decided, once again, to go vegetarian. I did this for several reasons: One, meat production is bad for the environment and for the animals who are living in horrible conditions in factory farms. Two, organic meat is substantially healthier than conventional meat, but it costs so much more. Three, I don't like meat. Four, eating meatless is significantly cheaper than eating meat.

"Going vegetarian really didn't have a lot to do with my diabetes. I haven't seen any difference in my sugars when eating meat and not eating meat. The key is to get enough protein, not necessarily enough protein from meat. However, many vegetarians consume too many carbs which isn't healthy for anyone's blood sugar. I have to make sure to get enough protein in my diet from nonmeat foods such as organic eggs, organic cheese, beans, and soy products like tofu and edamame.

"My girls (ages three and one) are both vegetarians like me. I do prepare meat sometimes, especially when we have guests coming over and for my husband who still consumes meat. However, I purchase organic meat for these occasions. We can afford to do so because we rarely purchase meat, so we save a lot on groceries in this regard.

"Whatever I make for dinner (and I am the primary chef in the family), they eat. I don't make two meals. Since my girls have never really had meat, except on rare occasions, they don't ask for meat.

"Almost anything can be made vegetarian—pizza, chili, soup, stir-fry, casseroles, and so on. Tofu is a tasteless protein that can be added to so many recipes. It takes on the flavor of what you are cooking. We even add tofu to our smoothies! I also make tofu banana bread. The tofu makes the bread dense and moist—yum! Not a tofu fan? There are plenty of other vegetarian protein options including cheese, beans, and eggs."

Catherine Vancak's first undergraduate degree was in ballet and food and nutrition. She says she got an excellent education on topics such as food science, childhood obesity, and vegetarianism. "I felt like I had the tools and knowledge to become a vegetarian. I did it because I thought it was a healthier choice and because of animal welfare. It actually went very well for quite a while. I was never deficient in vitamins or experienced a lag in energy.

"Then I was diagnosed with type 1 diabetes. I remained a vegetarian for one year after. After reading a few books on low-carb diets, I thought it would make managing my diabetes a little easier if I replaced foods that were higher in carbohydrates like cottage cheese or Greek yogurt with meat. Reluctantly, I started eating meat again and saw an improvement in my blood sugars. Currently I live close to a Whole Foods, so I can get organic meats that make me feel a little better about consuming meat.

"I certainly think that it's possible for a woman with diabetes to be a vegetarian. It requires a lot of planning, but then again diabetes in general requires a lot of planning! My best advice would be to spread your carbohydrate intake throughout the day so that meal time boluses don't get too large and unpredictable."

Q&A WITH CLAIRE M. BLUM, MSEd, RN, CDE

Claire is program coordinator for Partners & Peers for Diabetes Care, Inc., and has lived with type 1 diabetes for thirty-four years.

The vegan diet is considered one of the best for people with diabetes. Tell me why you decided to start following a vegan diet. Blood sugar control? Weight loss? Ethical issues?

Vegan eating has always been a way of life for me, as my parents became very health conscious around the time I was born. When I grew older I began adding dairy and eggs to my diet, back in the days when it was pretty difficult to find healthy vegetarian, let alone vegan, options on the go. This allowed for flexibility in cooking and I enjoyed the textures and taste that dairy and eggs provided. Now in my later years, since discovering that I have numerous food sensitivities, it has become necessary to eliminate dairy and eggs from my diet again. I've always believed that eating a vegetarian diet has contributed to my health and well-being. Serious weight gain has never been an issue in my life, and my endocrinologist tells me that I will never die of heart disease!

Tell me about your diet. How do you get enough protein as a vegan?

My diet is very simple, consisting mostly of whole grains, nuts, seeds, veggies, fruits, and healthy oils. Food as close to its natural goodness as possible … where all the nutrients are safely hidden and stored. In recent years, I've had to forego the legumes, as they seem to pose problems for my digestive system, but with mindful eating, I am still able to get adequate protein. Many people worry that eating a vegan or vegetarian diet will not provide adequate protein, without realizing that any combination of whole grains, nuts and seeds, or legumes, contains all the amino acids necessary for a complete protein.

Do you feel like the vegan diet is sustainable over the long term?

Nowadays it is pretty easy to eat vegan, because there are so many health food stores and restaurants that cater to the vegetarian/vegan lifestyle. Really, it's all about learning how to cook and enjoy foods in their natural state, and enjoying the added benefit of health and well-being!

Have you found a reduced need for insulin with a vegan diet?

My insulin need ranges BETWEEN 25 and 28 units per day, which is pretty good considering that I eat a lot of whole grain "carbs."

What advice would you give to someone wanting to switch to a vegan diet?

When your body gets the nutrition it needs, you feel better, and have fewer cravings for unhealthy foods!

An excellent resource is The Physicians Committee for Responsible Medicine, with well-researched support, recipes, and menus for use of a vegan diet with diabetes. http://pcrm.org/health/diabetes-resources/

AUTHENTIC ADVICE

■ *Eating right with diabetes can seem like a game without rules but by knowing the food you're eating, it puts you back in control. You are eating for you, nobody else! Always test your blood sugar and take the time to check in with how your body is feeling. There are fewer surprises that way. It sounds simple*

(continued)

AUTHENTIC ADVICE (continued)

but it's surprising how much we miss when we're not looking. ■ Catherine Vancak

■ If someone wants to try a vegetarian diet, go "flexitarian" (part-time vegetarian). Watch how you feel better and consume more healthy foods (fruits, veggies, whole grains, vegetarian proteins). Additionally, you should see a drop in your grocery bill, which is crucial for many in the current economy. Do your research. There are thousands of vegetarian recipes available. I would also recommend speaking with a dietitian to make sure you are getting enough protein in your diet. A diet full of carbohydrates and no protein isn't healthy for one's blood sugars or one's weight. ■ Rachel Garlinghouse

7   High Maintenance Holidays

I've been a high maintenance eater for as long as I can remember. I think my parents would say I was fairly high maintenance even before I was diagnosed with diabetes at fourteen years old. I've never liked to try new foods and mostly stick to what I like. Living with diabetes, routine makes my life easier, which is all fine and good 90 percent of the time. I cook dinner for my family almost every night and eat almost all of my meals at home, and that way, I eat what I like and my blood sugars stay relatively stable.

It's the holidays that screw me up.

From Thanksgiving to New Year's Eve there will be dinners out and parties and various celebrations, and for all these years that I've lived with diabetes, I always end up with high and low blood sugars during the holidays. I will eat the exact same meal at my mom's house that I would prepare at my own, and somehow, after dinner I'll be low. It has made me careful when it comes to what I put on my plate, but a side effect of being "careful" is that I feel high maintenance. "You don't like mashed potatoes?" someone will ask, and it makes me want to scream. *Of course* I like mashed potatoes, I *love* mashed potatoes, but I can't eat them. Someone else will say, "Aren't you going to have some of the pumpkin pie?" It's the same thing every year.

Most of my family understands my eating habits and it's only when there are new guests at the table that these questions are asked. And of course the holidays are only a few days out of the year; I can have some pie and an extra bolus to cover the delicious dessert if I want to, but most of the time it's not worth the trouble.

This time I've decided to take a new approach. From here on out I'm going to think about the way I eat not as high maintenance, but as taking care of myself. It's a lot easier than it was years ago thanks to the wide variety of Atkins dieters, vegans, Paleo, and low carbers out there who help me feel less alone when it comes to eating thoughtfully. So, with the swarms of specialized eaters out there, I'm going to embrace my high maintenance self and hold my head high when I explain that no, I'm not eating any mashed potatoes. Pass me the brussels sprouts instead.

Special events and holidays can be particularly challenging for people with diabetes. For example, my extended family had a large gathering at Easter earlier this month and dinner was served at 3 pm. I wasn't hungry at 3 pm. I'd eaten lunch at 12 because I was hungry at 12, and so I sat at the table with my family feeling high maintenance. This wasn't our normal family holiday routine, but this sort of thing has happened to me periodically as a woman with diabetes.

So how do we manage to eat right when it comes to holidays, special events, and various stages of our lives? Susan Weiner, RD, MS, CDE, CDN, says people with diabetes often feel overwhelmed when they are first diagnosed with the disease. "As an RD, CDE, I work with people who have type 1 and type 2 diabetes. People with diabetes benefit from nutritional counseling because they often require guidance on how to best control blood sugar levels with proper nutrition. Meal planning should be a coordinated effort between the person with diabetes, or their parent or caregiver, and an RD, CDE. That way food preferences can be incorporated into the meal plan, which will increase long-term compliance. If you're not happy with what you're eating, you won't continue to eat well. So, nutritional counseling can help improve long-term blood sugar control and possibly prevent or delay diabetes complications."

When it comes to holidays and special events, Weiner says pre-planning can be very helpful. "It's important to enjoy family holidays and special functions. It's not all about the food. What do

Easter and other holidays mean to you besides food? Do you love the traditional stories? Do you see people/family/friends you don't ordinarily see during the year? Please don't make the holidays only about food."

Alyssa Rosenzweig says she has learned to navigate through social situations and special celebrations. "My immediate family and friends are the least understanding when it comes to eating. My dad loves to go to restaurants to celebrate any occasion," she says. "When I was younger everyone wanted to take me out to dinner for my birthday and my dad would get frustrated when I didn't want to go. It always felt like I was breaking family traditions and letting people down." She says that she loves to cook and chooses to: "I put love and passion into a meal."

Alyssa also says that dating is hard because the most typical date is to go out to dinner. "I don't want to make it seem like I don't appreciate the gesture," she says. When she asked a friend for advice he said to slowly let people know how it works and that finding good foods to cook and eat together can be a positive challenge to the budding relationship.

TIPS

In her expert column on the Diabetes Sisters website, Jennifer Stallings, RD, LDN, CDE, CPT, offers tips on managing a good diet during the holidays.

- Always make sure there are healthy choices available in addition to more traditional foods. That way you can eat high fiber veggies and smaller portions of your favorite foods.
- Focus on the people instead of the food.
- Don't deprive yourself.

(continued)

TIPS (*continued*)

■ Try to stay physically active throughout the holidays. You'll feel better and have more energy. And it will balance off some of those extra treats, whether your chief concern is blood sugar control, weight management, or both.

■ Keep your appetite under control. Skipping breakfast in preparation for the office potluck leaves you so hungry that you could overdo it. Instead, eat regular meals that include carb, protein, and a little fat. It spreads food throughout the day and keeps your appetite and blood sugars controlled.

■ Balance holiday treats with lower fat, lower carb foods instead of filling up on only "goodies." Turkey with the stuffing, raw veggies with the real mashed potatoes, green salad with the fruit ambrosia. This works on your own plate and when planning a holiday menu. Every dish does not have to be a major production.

■ Learn the carb values of the holiday foods you love. Make a plan to fit them in, so you do not feel deprived on the holidays. Remember it's a give and take when it comes to the meal plan.

■ Think about your choices. When offered a high fat or high carb holiday treat, consider whether you really want it. Are you hungry? Is it something you love? Or would you just be eating it because it's there? If you save those choices for the things you really love, it will help keep things merry and moderate.

■ If your chief concern is weight or you must limit the amount of carb eaten at a meal to keep your blood sugars under control, use the "plate method." Set aside half the plate for salad and vegetables. Use about a quarter for protein foods and the rest for carbs.

- At a buffet, preview the whole thing before making any choices. This helps you fit in the things you want most instead of already having a plateful when you see something you really want.
- Drink lots of water. It's filling and good for you.

Lesley Hoffman Goldenberg says, "Yes! Being Jewish is fulfilling and wonderful, but there are so many challenges being a type 1 diabetic Jewish woman! Meals are often carb heavy when they are for special holidays. Most holidays start with a big, thick, and delicious challah bread and have multiple courses with lots of talking and eating. I've never felt pressure to eat or forced to eat something, but there is always TONS of food at holiday meals, which makes it very difficult to accurately count everything.

"Ironically, I used to keep kosher but found it healthier not to keep kosher. For me, it became so much easier and healthier to dine out in a restaurant and order a piece of non-kosher chicken with a side dish instead of ordering a heavier lasagna, pasta, or even a dense carb-filled veggie burger. I eventually stopped keeping kosher to offer myself more flexibility and healthier options. I'll add the disclaimer that there are plenty of diabetics who also keep kosher and they make it work for them; it was just too challenging for me."

DINING OUT

After I was diagnosed I used to hate going out to dinner because somehow, no matter what I did, my blood sugars would be too high or too low. I hated having to sneak off to the bathroom to give my shot. There were also those times when I gave my shot and the dinner took forever to arrive, and I would be eating skittles at the table while we waited for our meal. Of course the pump makes everything easier for me, but going out to dinner will always be a challenge.

Riva Greenberg says she used to sneak off to the ladies room to take her pre-meal injection. "But after years of dimly lit rooms and stalls, nowhere to balance your pocket book, vial, and meter, feeling like a criminal hiding some dirty deed, I decided no more lurking or skurking. I shoot up at the dinner table now—and the funniest thing is no one ever seems to notice. Of course I've become pretty talented at measuring out my dose and injecting without drawing attention to myself. I can even do it in the middle seat of an airplane!"

Rachel Garlinghouse says her family rarely dines out because of the cost, "and because I think homemade food tastes better. However, when we do eat out, I am very careful about what I eat. Sometimes I'll look up the food's nutritional facts online before we leave. I'm not afraid to order something to my exact preferences or send food back if it doesn't match the order. Usually I find it helpful to tell the server, if applicable, that I'm diabetic. They tend to perk up and take extra care of our family. I have, on occasion, been low while dining out. I tell the server I'm diabetic and ask for a small cup of soda or juice."

Aliza Chana Zaleon hates checking her blood glucose in front of people, "but on the other hand, it increases awareness at times and can spark great discussions. There are just times, though, that I want an evening to relax with my family and not be 'on' as the advocate, and not have to worry about what others around me will think about someone checking blood glucose at the dinner table. If I'm low, I am always downing Smarties, having to answer questions, and wonder if I will go into 'dumping syndrome' because I have gastroparesis. I'm pretty good at carb counting and I'm on the pump, so if I'm high, I can temporarily increase my bolus. The pump is also great for being able to completely suspend insulin, but if there is insulin on board and I'm low, there isn't much that can be done but ask for a sugared soda or juice."

Sysy Morales says, "When I eat out, I usually do low carb so that I don't have to worry about large amounts of insulin in such a public setting. I take shots and have noticed how looking at people and smiling while injecting discreetly in my abdomen seems to put them at ease."

Before Linda Frick went on the pump she says it was incredibly tricky to be able to eat late at a restaurant without suffering from a low. "If there was bread or chips I would nibble on that before my dinner came. Sometimes I would wait until after the meal to give my shot since there was nothing worse than ruining a meal with a low blood sugar problem! There were occasions where I was so low that I couldn't order without confusion and my husband would need to 'take over' and do it for me and then slip me some candy. Probably like most diabetics, when I get really low, I often will get stubborn and lose my taste for most everything. Now that I'm older and on the pump, when I go out to eat, I often will steer clear of lots of carbs and opt for more healthy eating by substituting veggies for potatoes, and so on, which means that I do test before I eat to keep from having to deal with any blood sugar issues. Now that glucometers are so small, I can easily test wherever and whenever I need to without a big hassle. It's almost impossible to gauge the exact carb content of many foods at restaurants, and they often use lots of fats in their meals, which will affect my blood sugar slowly. I will usually guesstimate my insulin needs based on previous experience and then keep retesting and readjusting with an insulin bolus. The only negative about eating out and being diabetic is that since the portion size is so large when you eat out, I always feel like I eat way too much and ultimately will need to take an extended bolus to cover the meal, especially if it's a large steak. Of course, I eat the whole thing!"

From the mashed potatoes at Thanksgiving to the chocolate at Valentine's Day, holidays are a challenge for people with diabetes. Says Riva Greenberg, "It's taken a long time but I no longer indulge in 'vacation or holiday eating.' You know, those times you say to yourself, well, it's okay to have whatever I want because I'm on vacation or it's the holidays. I don't really know how or why, but I reached a place where I want to be healthy and taking a big excursion from that doesn't give me joy. This week I met a group of friends and one had arranged for us to do something a little different: a food tour in NYC. It took place in Greenwich Village, in the Italian section that still hums with great pizza, bakeries, and pork and cheese shops. Our tour began with pizza and went on to include rice balls, another type of pizza, olive oil on Italian bread, a big buttery chocolate chip cookie, and ended with a cannoli. At first I felt a little bummed that most of the food on the tour I wouldn't usually eat and don't really eat anymore. Then I just decided to enjoy my friends' company and the historic part of the tour and have a couple of bites of pizza, enjoy the cheese and salami, give the cookie to my husband and the cannoli to someone else. But generally, during the holidays when there are tempting foods around, I don't usually eat. I will have a few bites and make sure that the next day I'm back to healthy eating and my one hour power walk. I really believe and live by the rule that you can have anything. Just have a little, now and then, and most of the time eat healthy and move."

Rachel Garlinghouse says the hardest part of the holidays is that they just keep going! "They really start at Halloween all the way through Easter. The best tip I read on watching what you eat is this—check out all the food options first. What do you really want the most? Eat sensibly for the most part and indulge on what you really want. Don't heap your plate with food that you could take or leave. I prefer to 'save my carbs' for the thing I can't live without—a slice of pumpkin pie or my mom's sugar knot bread rolls.

"All my family members and friends know I'm diabetic, so I am never hounded about trying foods. Additionally, I'm a vegetarian. My family has been great about making sure there are some vegetarian, low-carb options at meals. I always bring a dish or two or three to contribute. My goal isn't to hinder anyone else's meal, nor is it to compromise my blood sugars."

Sysy Morales, who has a younger sister with type 1, says, "My parents have been eating healthier these past few years and serve plenty of healthy dishes at the holidays in an effort to support everyone's health. It's all about great tasting food and health and wellness for everyone! In the past, I've had to politely decline food from people. They don't always like it, but I always try to explain to them why I'm declining their delicious food and if they don't understand I know any disappointment on their part isn't my problem. It's not fun but the 'please people at any costs' stage of my life is over."

Linda Frick doesn't get stressed about eating during the holidays. "I splurge, bolus, splurge, bolus, and splurge!! It's only a day or two so nothing to get worked up over. If my blood sugar goes high, I know how to fix it. Since I've had diabetes for so long, I will often feel ill if I eat things that I should stay away from. So with that in mind, my eating of holiday sweets just only lasts a day and then I'm over it completely until the next holiday.

"When I was younger, I was very affected by my friends' and coworkers' disapproval of things that I was eating. It actually turned me into a closet eater in my younger years. My mother, however, was very supportive of my restrictions and almost always had a 'sugar free' homemade dessert for me for certain occasions like Christmas, birthdays, and Thanksgiving. Now that I'm older and more opinionated and brazen about myself, I could care less about what others think or say about what I eat and I'm always looking for an opportunity to 'educate.' I find that most people still think of diabetic care like they did forty years ago. A lot has changed since then."

Cultural Traditions

When my husband and I want to go out to eat, I'll scan through the local guide to read about the various restaurant offerings we have here in South Carolina, and often wonder what it means when a restaurant is described as "American." Burgers and fries? Meatloaf? Apple pie? What is American food, and do I want to eat it? Whether we live in the North, South, East, or West, we all are a part of the big American melting pot and most of us can choose to eat Italian,

French, Greek, Indian, Chinese, or American food every night of the week. Some of these foods are better than others when it comes to eating right with diabetes, which can pose a problem for those people firmly entrenched in those cultures.

Rachel Garlinghouse thinks that the American diet is centered around meat. "Being a vegetarian means that my girls and I have to eat around the main dish. However, there are so many fabulous side dishes—many of them veggies—that we don't mind at all!"

Aliza Chana Zaleon keeps kosher, which she feels is more carb-heavy. "Passover, anyone? Latkes on Chanukah? But these are once a year 'treats' and then they are done! So, I am allowed my matzoh on Passover, the special 'death by chocolate cake' that my mom makes only on Passover, and the latkes on the first night of Chanukah and one other night when we have family and friends come over for a Chanukah party. Other than that, I'm done."

Katie Peterson is a graduate student at Boston University, but in 2010 when she was 26 years old, she was incorrectly diagnosed with type 2 diabetes. "While I started taking Metformin, which made me really sick, I refused to pick up the meter the doctor had prescribed me (although had not taught me how to use). Luckily, through my own research, I found an endocrinologist who I met with about a week later. He was fantastic from day one, spending more than an hour talking with me and finally giving me the support I needed. He taught me how to monitor my blood glucose and talked some sense into me about the importance of doing it. He also did further blood tests, which suggested I have latent autoimmune diabetes in adults—type 1.5 diabetes.

"For the past two years, I have been able to manage my diabetes through a combination of oral medications, a strict diet, and exercise. However, since it appears that I have a type of slow onset type 1, at some point I likely will have to move to insulin therapy."

One of the things that drew Katie to her graduate program is her fascination with humans' relationship with food. As she puts it, "Food is often overlooked as something to study because it is such a necessity—so everyday. But I find the way people relate to and identify themselves through food to be an extremely interesting subject area.

"The relationship with food is even more complex for people with diabetes. Thinking about food is constant—from counting the carbs of everything consumed to guessing how something will affect blood glucose. For those with diabetes, food can fluctuate between being seen as the savior and the enemy depending on the latest blood glucose reading.

"Because of my interest in the relationship people with diabetes have with food, I decided to study this area further in one of my classes last semester. My research focused on how cultural food identity, or how people identify themselves culturally through their food choices, affects the management of type 2 diabetes.

"I read through study after study that discussed how people with type 2 diabetes struggled to change their diets after diagnosis because the health professionals they were working with did not take their culture into consideration when offering nutritional advice. Too often the health professionals did not understand the patients' cultural background or did not think about it when discussing dietary options. Because culture influences everything, from the ingredients someone uses to the way they prepare and consume food, however, this is crucial.

"I discovered a couple of successful type 2 diabetes pilot programs, including one on the southern border of Texas and one in rural South Carolina, that were designed to fit the needs of the specific communities. Every aspect of each program was developed based on the participants' culture. For example, when talking about food the health professionals used food items and ingredients that the participants were accustomed to and presented cooking demonstrations of healthier versions of traditional dishes. This focus on culture had an extremely positive impact. The pilot program participants had much more success improving their dietary behaviors and lowering their A1Cs than those in traditional programs."

In her paper for school, "When Culture and Health Collide: Examining the Role of Cultural Food Identity in Type 2 Diabetes Nutrition Education Programs," Katie concluded that when faced with a diagnosis of type 2 diabetes, it is "extremely difficult to make significant dietary changes, especially ones that seem to be in conflict with one's cultural food choices." In this report she examined the effectiveness of programs that address the importance of working within cultural eating patterns when trying to change and improve a diabetic's diet. Katie looked at a program in South Carolina called the Soul Food Light, developed for African Americans with type 2 diabetes in rural South Carolina. According to the study:

> *In Black cultural traditions, meals are social events with friends and family. Therefore, a traditional African American meal prepared with low-fat techniques and ingredients was served to participants and family members following most classes. Meals were framed as social events, such as a church homecoming supper or Fourth of July picnic. Participation of family members was encouraged not only to integrate Black cultural traditions associated with food but also to capitalize on the value of family and to provide transportation, a common barrier in rural areas.*
>
> *These meals provided hands-on learning opportunities as participants helped with meal preparation, discussed ingredients, and learned how to read food labels. When the educational sessions had been completed, participants took part in discussion groups facilitated by a nurse who was a certified diabetes educator. The discussions focused on nutrition and participants were encouraged to share their experiences and struggles with food. Weekly follow-up telephone calls with a nurse also provided participants the opportunity to discuss successes and challenges, as well as ask questions.*

Katie only looked at the role of cultural identity and food in people with type 2, but says that some of her findings definitely apply to people with type 1. "For example, one of the major themes in my findings was how important it is for the health community to take patients' culture into consideration when offering nutritional advice. So many people who have been diagnosed with diabetes are told they have to change the way they eat, but the way someone eats is often so closely aligned with their cultural identity that it can be nearly impossible. The health community needs to do a better job of understanding patients' cultures so that they can offer dietary solutions that are relevant.

"There are many cultures where certain ingredients, preparation techniques, and commensality are key to identity, but the health community has often ignored this. I discussed a study on British Pakistani Muslims that is a perfect example of this. Their doctors told them to eat foods that were completely foreign to them, which resulted in them feeling like they had to give up their traditional foods and by extension, their cultural identity, in order to manage their diabetes. Instead, the doctors should have focused on helping these patients make changes that fit with their culture, such as making lighter versions of traditional dishes and reducing portion size. I also looked at a couple of pilot programs that took this approach and the results were incredible. When people feel like they are understood culturally, and are given tools to make dietary changes in a way that doesn't conflict with their identity, they are much more likely to have success managing diabetes.

"I've definitely grown more aware of just how complex the relationship with food is for people with diabetes. In my studies, I've looked a lot at how things like culture, identity, and socioeconomics play into how people think and feel about food. These thoughts and feelings are that much more complicated when a chronic illness that is so centered on food is involved."

Alcohol and Celebrations

The American Diabetes Association (ADA) recommends "practicing caution" when it comes to drinking alcohol. The ADA website states:

Alcohol can cause hypoglycemia shortly after drinking and for 24 hours after drinking. So, if you want to drink alcohol, check your blood glucose before you drink and eat either before or while you drink. You should also check your blood glucose before you go to bed to make sure it is at a safe level—between 100 and 140 mg/dL. If your blood glucose is low, eat something to raise it.

MORE TIPS TO SIP BY

- Drink only when and if blood glucose is under control. Do not omit food from your regular meal plan.
- Test blood glucose to help you decide if you should drink.
- Wear an I.D. that notes you have diabetes.
- Sip a drink slowly to make it last.
- Have a no-calorie beverage by your side to quench your thirst.
- Try wine spritzers to decrease the amount of wine in the drink.
- Use calorie-free drink mixers: diet soda, club soda, diet tonic water, or water.
- Drink alcohol with a snack or meal. Some good snack ideas are pretzels, popcorn, crackers, fat-free or baked chips, raw vegetables, and a low-fat yogurt dip.
- Find a registered dietitian to help you fit alcohol into your food plan.
- Do not drive or plan to drive for several hours after you drink alcohol.

Rachel Garlinghouse says, "Neither of our families drink alcohol, so it isn't part of our celebrations. However, Steve and I do drink a glass of wine on occasion, and I usually have it every night, about one week out of the month, when my sugars tend to spike. Dry red wine is not only healthy, but it suppresses glycogen release, helping me manage my sugars."

Sysy Morales and her husband drink liquor for different occasions. "We stick to one or two shots only, straight up, and focus on the taste of the liquor versus it's affect from alcohol. We try to focus on what we're celebrating and keep in mind that even if I didn't have diabetes, we're still the parents of two young children and neither of us wants to drink too much alcohol, anyway. We stick with liquor because I know how much insulin I need for it, versus some mixed drink."

I like to have a glass of red wine just about every night. Drinking has been a tradition on both sides of my family, with good results and bad. Some family members are self-described alcoholics who follow AA and no longer drink, while others, like my husband and me, enjoy a glass of wine in the evenings as a form of relaxation. Red wine has proven heart-healthy benefits and like everything, as long as it's consumed in moderation, it can be a part of a healthy lifestyle.

In her *Diabetes Self-Management* blog, Amy Campbell, CDE, RD, LDN, writes that there are no hard and fast rules when it comes to drinking alcohol. *"That's why I repeatedly state that it's important to have this discussion with your health care provider, as the 'rules' can vary from person to person."*

Fitting Alcohol into Your Meal Plan

Alcohol is unlike carbohydrate, protein, and fat. However, alcohol is metabolized, or handled, by the body in a manner similar to fat. This means that calories from alcohol can easily be stored as fat unless you burn them off. Alcohol contains 7 calories per gram; fat contains 9 calories per gram, and carb and protein contain 4 calories per gram. So alcohol is a prime source of calories. If you're trying to lose or maintain your weight, you need to think about this carefully. An occasional glass of wine isn't a problem. But if you tend to have a glass of wine every night, you need to consider that 4 ounces of wine contains about 90 calories. Over time, this can add up. You may want to cut out 90 calories somewhere else in your meal plan to balance things out and avoid that spare tire around your waist.

Remember, too, that alcohol may lead to low blood glucose in people taking insulin with a meal or those taking a sulfonylurea drug, such as glipizide, glyburide, or glimepiride. If you take any of these types of medicines, be sure to eat a carbohydrate-containing food, such as bread, pasta, rice, or fruit, with your alcohol. If you need to shave calories from somewhere else in your meal plan, you may want to think about cutting out some fat, such as margarine, oil, or salad dressing, for example.

How Much to Drink?

To best answer this question, it helps to know serving sizes of common alcoholic beverages. All of these are considered a serving: 5 ounces of red or white wine; 12 ounces of beer; 1½ ounces (a shot glass) of distilled spirits (such as vodka, rum, or whiskey).

Men are "allowed" more alcohol than women because men can process alcohol more efficiently. Therefore, if and when you choose to drink, the guideline for men is no more than two servings of alcohol per day; for women, no more than one serving.

Best Choices

Things can be as murky as a mudslide when it comes to deciding *what* to drink. The "best" choices, though, are those that don't contain too many calories or carbs. Try dry white or red wine or champagne, light beer, or distilled spirits. Fruity drinks, such as piña coladas, daiquiris, and margaritas contain fruit juices and therefore contain more calories and carbs. In fact, 4 ounces of a strawberry daiquiri can contain 200 calories and 30 grams of carbs or more. And many people don't stop at just one! Stouts and ales (think Guinness or Sam Adams lager) approach 200 calories per 12-ounce bottle. More of a gin and tonic or rum and coke lover? Go for diet tonic water and diet soda as your mixers. If you drink alcoholic beverages that contain a significant amount of carbohydrate, talk to your dietitian or health care provider about how to fit these into your eating plan safely.

What about nonalcoholic beer and wine? Because these beverages contain little, if any, alcohol, you may actually need to count them as carbohydrate choices in your meal plan. Many nonalcoholic beers contain close to 15 grams of carb which is equal to one slice of bread or one small piece of fruit.

Desserts

What about desserts? Do we indulge or not? Can we have just one bite of cake or is it too hard to stop there? Do we have to look the other way when others are having their cake and eating it, too? I am a big fan of dark chocolate, which to me is one of those items I would request if I was playing the "stuck on a desert island" game: red wine, dark chocolate, peanut butter (I almost forgot coffee!) and a book. On those rare occasions that my husband and I go out to dinner, I often wish restaurants would offer a bar of dark chocolate on the dessert menu. I wouldn't eat the whole thing, of course, but just a square or two to satisfy that sweet craving. Dark chocolate, like red wine and coffee, has benefits for people with diabetes. An ounce of dark chocolate has approximately 130 calories, 10 grams of fat, 6 grams of saturated fat, and 15 grams of carbohydrate. Studies have shown health benefits like insulin sensitivity, anti-inflammatory, and hypertension reductions. Flavanols, which are found in berries, apples, grape juice, wine, and cocoa, have health benefits. The less processing the cocoa is subject to, the higher the levels of flavanols. The highest levels of flavanols are found in cocoa. Amy Campbell suggests choosing a dark chocolate with a cocoa content higher than 50 percent and main ingredients of cocoa butter and cocoa solids.

Rachel Garlinghouse loves dessert. "I have always enjoyed baking, so I have learned ways to lower the carb count of my desserts without compromising the flavor or texture. Indulge? Always! But again, I enjoy with purpose. If I know an array of desserts will be offered, I eat a veggie-filled meal with some protein first."

Sysy Morales likes dessert and tries to be a little picky. "If someone is offering me one of my favorite desserts, I'll have a few bites and then share or give away the rest. If what is offered is not one of my favorites, I prefer sticking to the blood sugar I'm having at the moment instead of risking it."

Linda Frick says: "Lets face it! Who doesn't love sweets? I do well managing a huge bite of something like pie or cookies but rarely will eat the whole thing since I don't want to feel poorly afterward. The exception to this is my addiction to cheesecake. I won't go out and buy one, but if it's on the table, I have difficulty saying no. I love that stuff! If I bolus enough I can and will do ok but with anything that fatty and sweet, it will take a toll on my ability to feel good afterward. I've learned over my years of being diabetic that I have favorite things and will only eat those things, which are far and few between. For instance a sourdough roll versus corn on the cob. I'd much rather have a roll than corn but the carbs are similar. Same for sweets. I'd never eat a doughnut but adore my cheesecake. I have to be a choosy consumer."

AUTHENTIC ADVICE

■ When it comes to the holidays, *I try to focus on activities and people during the holidays. This means that I end up forgetting about food a little and find that helps. For the feasts, I pick out what I really want to have and try to keep portions small.*
■ Sysy Morales

■ *I would encourage people with diabetes to have the confidence to speak openly with their health team about food. Just as it is important for the health community to understand patients' cultural backgrounds, it is important that patients push for information that relates to their culture. If a doctor or nutritionist offers you advice that you know you won't follow, speak up and ask for alternatives. Tell them about the foods you eat, and ask for help making small changes that can lead to better blood glucose control. The more your health team knows about your food culture, the better equipped they will be to offer culturally sensitive help. I would also encourage people with diabetes to do their own research and find ways to tweak their favorite recipes.* ■ Katie Peterson

■ *Desserts in moderation. Nothing is forbidden and nothing in excess. Moderation is key.* ■ Aliza Chana Zaleon

■ *Diabetes throughout the life cycle should be individually managed. No two people are the same. Individualized meal plans and food preferences should always be considered.*
■ Susan Weiner

8   Tummy Troubles: Diabetes and Digestive Issues

People with diabetes are frequently diagnosed with digestive problems such as celiac disease, thyroid issues, gluten intolerance, and gastroparesis. While my digestion is healthy now, I am always on the lookout for problems because I know as a woman with type 1 diabetes, I am at an increased risk. But who wants to talk about indigestion, gas, diarrhea, and bloating? Gross! It wasn't until I became a mother (and was changing poopy diapers, getting thrown up on, and wiping bums on a regular basis) that I was able to talk about "tummy" issues with my husband, and even now, we keep it to a minimum! Grossness aside, and in the words from my toddler's favorite book, *Everyone Poops*. Even us women with diabetes. And when things are not working correctly, it can be painful and debilitating. So why do we wait to get help?

Studies show that these digestive issues are underdiagnosed, and in my humble opinion there are a variety of nonscientific reasons for a delayed diagnosis. First, it's because no one wants to go to the doctor and talk about pooping problems. I can barely bring myself to talk about my period or sex with the doctor, and maybe I'm the only private one out there, but I think talking about intimate issues with your doctor is never easy. And change is hard. Everyone has a friend who is *gluten-intolerant*, and we've all heard about how hard it is to cook, shop, pay for, and eat on a gluten-free diet. As women with diabetes, we are restricted enough with what we can eat, and none of us wants to discover that we have even fewer food options to choose from. Finally, I think that another reason that digestive problems are underdiagnosed is because one of the symptoms is weight loss. If a woman is losing weight as a result of gas and bloating, it's tempting to ignore the problem. Is my stomachache really that bad, we might ask ourselves? While I no longer struggle with bulimia and work hard to eat healthy and exercise consistently, I will always be speaking from a disordered eating point of view. But I don't think it's a stretch to say that unexplained weight loss will not send women running to the doctor.

In Susan Weiner's expert opinion, part of the problem is that when you don't feel well for a long time, eating can become a comfort. "So women with undiagnosed celiac disease might reach for complex high-fiber carbohydrates, thus making celiac worse. I think the symptoms of celiac disease should be part of an assessment form for people with diabetes. Although many women might not have symptoms early on, at least they will be able to recognize the symptoms if they appear over time. As an RD, CDE, I work with people who have diabetes and celiac disease to develop a meal plan that fits all of their needs. By individualizing the meal plan, women will be much less overwhelmed. If a woman is a stay-at-home mom with three small children, the meal plan might be different than someone who commutes three hours each day to a job outside of the home. I LISTEN to my patients and clients. I don't suggest eating plans, which are too restrictive. It leads to unnecessary binging. We also explore mindful eating decisions." Susan recommends meeting with a registered dietitian who is also a certified diabetes educator. She says when you make the appointment, ask if the provider has knowledge about celiac disease. Not every RD, CDE is well versed in celiac disease.

No one wants to change her diet, but no one wants to live with pain either. In this chapter I've talked with a handful of women to understand these digestive issues and offer tips on living well with diabetes and digestive disorders.

CELIAC DISEASE, GLUTEN SENSITIVITY, OR GSE

Celiac disease is an autoimmune disorder triggered by gluten, a protein found in certain grains, which damages the small intestines and decreases its ability to absorb nutrients. People with type 1 diabetes, as well as those with other autoimmune conditions such as thyroid disease, are more at risk for celiac disease.

Amy Campbell, MS, RD, LDN, CDE, nutritionist at Joslin Diabetes Center and co-author of *16 Myths of a "Diabetic Diet"* writes about Celiac in her *Diabetes Self-Management* blog:

Facts and Figures

About three million people in the United States have celiac disease, but only 5 percent (150,000) are actually diagnosed. Twenty-five percent of new diagnoses occur in adults older than sixty years of age. And 6 percent of people with type 1 diabetes have celiac. In people with type 2 diabetes, about 1 in 250 have celiac. Having a family history of celiac increases the risk by between 5 percent and 15 percent. Celiac disease tends to be more common in people of European ancestry, as well as in people who have autoimmune diseases, including type 1 diabetes, lupus, rheumatoid arthritis, and autoimmune thyroid disease.

Symptoms

Gas
Bloating
Diarrhea
Weight loss
Lack of appetite
Fatigue, but some people do not experience any of the gastrointestinal symptoms.

Some less common symptoms include:

Anemia
Osteopenia (low bone density)
Fatty liver
Recurrent miscarriages
Short stature (in children)
Skin rash
Unexplained hypoglycemia

Diagnosis

Celiac disease is extremely underdiagnosed in the United States. A delay in diagnosis of celiac disease can increase the chance of developing other autoimmune diseases, along with increasing risk of osteoporosis, anemia, peripheral neuropathies, and some cancers. If you have type 1 diabetes and have any of these symptoms listed above, it is probably best to discuss this with your doctor. Celiac disease is diagnosed by a blood test that measures specific antibodies in your blood and if those are positive, then an intestinal biopsy is conducted to examine the small intestine and determine if there has been any damage.

Diagnosis of Celiac Disease

Celiac disease is diagnosed in a very specific manner. For a person to be diagnosed with this condition, at least three factors need to be in place.

First, a person must have either the HLA DQ2 or HLA DQ8 gene (don't worry; this won't turn into a genetics lesson!). This means that a person is genetically predisposed to getting celiac. Eating gluten-containing foods doesn't cause celiac.

Second, as with most autoimmune diseases, including type 1 diabetes, something needs to "trigger" the onset of celiac, such as an illness or infection, stress, surgery, puberty, pregnancy, etc.

And third, you must have been exposed to gluten in some form (which is pretty easy to do, given the number of foods that contain gluten).

According to the Gluten Intolerance Group, diagnosis of celiac starts with a blood test, which looks for high levels of certain kinds of antibodies. Blood tests don't confirm the diagnosis, however; the "gold standard" for diagnosis is a biopsy of the villi of the small intestine. A physician will do this by inserting a narrow, flexible tube down your throat into your small intestine, where a piece of the intestinal tissue is taken. If the biopsy indicates that you have flattened villi, in all likelihood, you have celiac. The final step in the diagnostic process is to go on a gluten-free diet for a period of time. If your symptoms improve, then it's highly probable that you have celiac.

It's important that people who suspect (or in whom their physician suspects) they might have celiac disease not go on a gluten-free diet before they are diagnosed. Otherwise, the biopsy may come out negative, and the person won't truly know if they have celiac or not.

Also, because celiac can run in the family, first-degree relatives (parents, siblings, or children) of the diagnosed person may also wish to be tested. About 5 percent to 15 percent of a person's first-degree relatives will have celiac.

Treatment

Treating celiac is pretty easy, yet can be awfully hard at the same time. At this point in time, the only treatment for celiac disease is to follow a gluten-free diet. A gluten-free diet must be followed for life. Gluten is a kind of protein found in wheat (including spelt, triticale, and Kamut), barley, and rye, and is what causes damage to the small intestine. This means that the obvious grain foods, such as bread, pizza crust, cereal, crackers, and pasta, for example, must be completely eliminated from the diet. On the positive side, though, there are many products that can be included in the diet, such as:

- *Rice*
- *Quinoa*
- *Amaranth*
- *Potato*
- *Buckwheat*
- *Corn*
- *Soy*
- *Bean flours*
- *Oats (with caution; if you do choose to eat oats, look for oats that are specifically labeled "gluten-free" as they can sometimes be cross-contaminated)*

This means that people with celiac disease can still eat bread, cereal, pasta, and crackers—as long as they're made with gluten-free ingredients such as those listed above.

Many grocery stores and natural food stores now sell gluten-free products, along with gluten-free flours, such as rice flour, so that you can bake your own bread and pizza crust, for example. Of course, you can still eat fruits, vegetables, lean protein foods, and healthy fats, such as olive oil. Dairy foods are okay, too, although you may have a temporary lactose intolerance due, to flattened villi (which usually resolves once the villi heal).

Most people with celiac will say that the hardest part about the diet isn't giving up regular bread or pasta; instead, it's knowing what's in the food that they eat. The tricky part about a gluten-free diet is that many processed and

packaged foods contain additives and other ingredients
that contain gluten. Wheat and wheat products are often
used as thickeners and stabilizers. Other foods may
contain modified food starch that contains gluten. One
must become an astute label reader and become very
familiar with acceptable ingredients. Even a tiny amount
of gluten is enough to cause damage to the intestine in
people with celiac.

For more of Amy's expertise on "Eating Right" with diabetes, check out her *Diabetes Self-Management* blog at www.diabetes-selfmanagement.com/blog/Amy-Campbell

Ginger Vieira has lived with type 1 diabetes and celiac disease for twelve years. She is a cognitive health coach, record-setting power-lifter, and author of *Your Diabetes Science Experiment*. I profiled Ginger as a "Smart Woman with Diabetes" on my blog and discovered that she diagnosed herself at the age of thirteen years old. She said, "The seventh grade in my middle school does an annual health fair. One of my classmates did his project on diabetes. I had all of the symptoms on his poster. My whole family had gotten the flu a few weeks earlier and it was like my flu just never went away. At first, no one believed me that I had diabetes, but I started crying a week later because I felt so awful, and my mom took me to the hospital.

"I spent three days in the hospital, and on the second day I started feeling really sorry for myself. I cried and cried whenever the doctors and nurses and my parents left the room. But that same day I started thinking about all of my friends, and everything they had already been through. I realized all of them had endured or continued to endure some immense challenges in their health, in their families, in life in general. And diabetes was simply one of my immense challenges. I left the hospital with that attitude, and left the self-pity behind."

Ginger started blogging in the diabetes community as a sophomore in college, and her main focus has always been in looking at the way people with diabetes think about the disease, and how that perspective impacts the way we live our lives.

"After two years of personal training, I knew that I loved supporting people in their goals to take care of their physical health, but I realized I wanted to support them in how they take care of their emotional health, too. In 2010, I enrolled in a cognitive-based coaching method (Results Coaches, from David Rock) that is based on the science of how our brains think about goals and obstacles, how to shape conversations to help someone understand themselves and their own goals better, and how to break down really overwhelming challenges and goals, and make them achievable.

"The phrase 'Living in Progress' comes quite simply from the fact that I believe the small steps we make every day toward our goals, toward becoming a better human being, toward learning how to live life to the fullest are the most important steps. The big steps that happen in our lives are really just the accumulation of all those little steps. We are constantly learning, and constantly making progress."

I checked back in with Ginger to ask her a few questions about living with celiac disease.

Q&A WITH GINGER VIEIRA

Studies show that women with diabetes have a higher risk of developing celiac disease, yet these women are often asymptomatic. Why is this, and what symptoms should women be aware of?

Celiac is so incredibly sneaky, that I suggest all the time that people get tested. Everything from your skin to your mood to your inability to sleep well can be related to celiac. People are sometimes scared to find out, and make the switch, but you feel so much better that the reward of knowing and getting gluten out of your body is sincerely worth it.

How is celiac diagnosed? What was your experience like? How long had you been feeling sick, and what made you go to your doctor?

I was very lucky. When I was fourteen, a year after my diabetes diagnosis, my endocrinologist had me check my celiac. I had virtually no symptoms aside from possible headaches, but still, they weren't severe enough that I really had any complaints. I was diagnosed so soon within the development of my celiac that very little damage was done to my small intestines.

Do you find that celiac affects your blood sugars?

Celiac on its own? No. What impacts my blood sugars is that following a gluten-free diet can mean you eat a very clean, low-carb diet. That being said, there's plenty of room for a person to eat a very junky diet while being gluten-free. When you're eating clean, and lower-carb, your diabetes will thank you. Today, I embrace my gluten-free life because I just feel excellent when I adhere to that style of nutrition.

I would imagine that a diagnosis of celiac in someone with diabetes would feel very overwhelming. We already have to follow a strict diet without digestive complications, so what can we do to help others feel less overwhelmed and what are some tips to help them maintain a gluten-free diet?

My biggest advice is to not think of what you can't eat anymore, but think of what your diet can now become. Celiac is the perfect motivator for getting all kinds of junk out of your diet. All that processed garbage will not be missed. Fill your nutrition plan with real veggies, fruit, lean meats, nuts, beans, and nutrition-packed grains like quinoa, and you will not miss gluten! There are so many great recipes for yummy treats like brownies and pancakes, but they'll be made with delicious whole-grain, gluten-free ingredients as opposed to overly processed white flour. Embrace this life. Once you get a hang of it, everything feels better and tastes better.

Ginger's enthusiasm is catching and she is a great role model for women with diabetes and celiac disease. For those who struggle to keep a positive attitude, below I discuss an article that addresses celiac and depression in women with diabetes. Being informed is an important coping mechanism to help women manage the stressors of living well with illness.

CELIAC AND DEPRESSION AND DISORDERED EATING

An article from *Diabetes Life* discusses the quadruple threat of diabetes digestive issues, depression, and disordered eating.

Women with celiac disease are more likely than the general population to report symptoms of depression and disordered eating, even when they adhere to a gluten-free diet, according to researchers at Penn State, Syracuse University, and Drexel University.

People with celiac disease often suffer from abdominal pain, constipation, decreased appetite, diarrhea, nausea, and vomiting in response to ingesting gluten. The disease affects somewhere between 1 in 105 to 1 in 1,750 people in the United States and is typically controlled by avoiding gluten-containing foods such as those made with wheat, barley, and rye.

> *It is easy to see how people who are not managing their disease well can frequently feel unwell and, therefore, be more stressed and have higher rates of depression, said Josh Smyth, professor of biobehavioral health and medicine at Penn State, But researchers had not carefully looked at whether people who are effectively managing celiac disease exhibit a greater risk for such difficulties.*

Smyth and his colleagues used a web-mediated survey to assess a range of physical, behavioral, and emotional experiences in

177 American women over the age of eighteen who reported a physician-provided diagnosis of celiac disease. The survey questions explored respondents' levels of adherence to a gluten-free diet and assessed various symptoms of celiac disease, how physical symptoms interfere with functioning, the respondents' experience and management of stressful situations, symptoms of clinical depression, and frequency of negative thoughts and behaviors associated with eating and body image.

We found that most participants frequently adhered to a gluten-free diet, and this greater compliance with diet was related to increased vitality, lower stress, decreased depressive symptoms and greater overall emotional health. However, even those people who were managing their illness very well reported higher rates of stress, depression, and a range of issues clustered around body dissatisfaction, weight, and shape when compared to the general population.

Smyth noted that he and his colleagues did not survey people without celiac disease; rather, they compared their results to those previously determined for the nonceliac population.

It is understandable to find that women with celiac disease tend to suffer from what is typically characterized as disordered eating, given that the focus of celiac-disease management is to pay careful attention to what and how one eats.

What we don't know is what leads to what and under what circumstances, he said. It's likely that the disease, stress, weight, shape and eating issues, and depression are interconnected. But we don't know if women with both higher stress and celiac disease are more likely to develop symptoms of disordered eating and then become depressed, or if women with celiac disease are depressed and then become stressed, which leads to disordered eating. In the future, we plan to investigate the temporal sequence of these symptoms.

The team's results may have implications for people with food allergies, diabetes, and Crohn's disease, a form of inflammatory bowel disease, as well as celiac disease, according to Smyth.

> *Going out to eat with friends or to a holiday potluck is a much different experience for these people because they have to be vigilant and monitor their diets. They may feel that they are a burden on a host or hostess. In many cases the only treatment option they are given is to manage their diets. I think we need to educate patients at diagnosis or post-diagnosis about some of the other associated difficulties they might experience and provide strategies for how to better manage those things. I am a proponent of elaborating our treatment models to not just address diseases, but also to address the psychological, social and behavioral aspects of disease as well, as they can influence disease outcomes and the well being of patients.*

Alyssa Rosenzweig was diagnosed with digestive issues soon after her diabetes diagnosis. At ten years old, that made eating feel very restricted. Gastroparesis runs in her family and she has to be careful about what she can eat. "In the last two years I've figured out what I can eat without worry and it's okay when I'm in my own world and can pack my lunch to take to work but it's harder when I'm traveling or when I go out to dinner. It's really hard to explain to people," she says. "I hate it when people say, 'What can't you eat?' It's easier to tell them what I CAN eat." Alyssa says gastroparesis is helped with exercise and that she swims or bikes every day. "The exercise gives me more forgiveness with food, digestion, and blood sugars."

Sysy Morales had digestive issues as a child before her diabetes diagnosis. "It was common for me to go to the pediatrician for constipation. I was given medication and sent on my way. About seven years after my diabetes diagnosis, at eighteen, I ended up in the hospital in severe pain with a bowel blockage. My diet up to this time revolved around dairy, wheat, corn, and animal protein. It was common for me to have frequent gas, bloating, abdominal pain, and nausea. Sometimes I'd throw up from the nausea. Doctors never gave me any tests or hinted that I should change my diet. They settled for my symptoms and attributed them to indigestion. Eventually, I spent years educating myself and learning about nutrition and health. I experimented more with food and kept a food diary.

"I have had a blood test for celiac and it came out negative. However, it seems I have gluten intolerance because if I eat it, I get gas, pain, bloating, constipation, and even acne. If I don't eat it, I'm completely void of those symptoms—even my skin clears up. It's a very dramatic difference and so I work to avoid grains. Sometimes I'll have birthday cake and sorely regret it the next day. Something that I really like to eat because it's gluten free and tasty and can replace rice in many recipes is the seed called quinoa. It's fast to cook, easy to find in most grocery stores now-a-days, and it's safe for me to eat.

"My favorite recipe with quinoa is for Quinoa Stuffed Peppers: This dish is fantastic as-is, but can easily be made vegetarian by completely omitting the ground beef. This really is a dish all in itself, so does not really need any accompaniments."

Sysy's Recipe For Quinoa Stuffed Peppers

Prep Time: 10 minutes
Cook Time: 40 minutes
Total Time: 50 minutes

Ingredients

2 large green bell peppers
1/2 pound ground sirloin
1 cup chopped onion
1/2 cup finely chopped carrot
1 clove garlic, finely minced
1 cup cooked quinoa
1 14 oz. can diced tomatoes

(continued)

Sysy's Recipe For Quinoa Stuffed Peppers (*continued*)

1/4 teaspoon salt
1/4 teaspoon ground black pepper
2 tablespoon finely chopped fresh basil
1/2 cup grated fresh parmesan cheese

Preparation

Preheat. the oven to 350°F.

Slice the green bell peppers in half vertically, and remove the pulp and seeds from the inside. Bring a large pot of salted water to a boil, and add the bell peppers. Boil for 5 minutes, then remove the peppers from the water, and set aside.

Heat a large skillet over medium-high heat, and add the hamburger. Break up the hamburger with a fork, and cook until the hamburger is no longer pink. Remove the hamburger, and set aside. Add the onion, carrot, and garlic to the pan, and cook 4–5 minutes, until vegetables are tender. Return the hamburger to the pan, and add the cooked quinoa, tomatoes, salt, and pepper. Continue cooking for 3–4 minutes, until heated through. Remove from the heat, and add the fresh basil.

Place the green pepper halves on a baking dish, and fill each cavity with about 3/4 cup of the quinoa mixture. Bake for 15 minutes.

Set the oven to the broil setting. Sprinkle the parmesan cheese evenly over the stuffed peppers, and broil for 2 minutes, until lightly browned.

Nikki Coar calls herself a glass-half-full type 1 diabetic who loves life. She says learning how to manage and live with diabetes was like taking a crash course in a foreign language. "Health providers would whip out terms to me like I was a seasoned veteran. To me, it might as well have been in Chinese. I had no idea what a 'bolus' was, and later didn't understand the difference between a bolus and a basal rate. And what the hell is 'background insulin'? What constituted a fast-acting insulin versus a slow-acting one? Can I really only have 30 carbs at breakfast and 45 at lunch and dinner? The nurses in the hospital took my BG regularly and would tell me my BG had gone from 300 to 185. Was that a good number? Where's it supposed to be at?" Nikki was diagnosed with celiac disease five months after her diabetes diagnosis and blogs at *Diabetes and Celiac Sunshine.*

Q&A WITH NIKKI COAR

Tell me about your diagnosis?

I diagnosed with type 1 diabetes on Saturday, February 6, 2010. The day before the Super Bowl. No one in my family has type 1 diabetes, so I was in complete disbelief.

Since the beginning of that week I'd felt like I had the stomach flu. When I woke up that Saturday, I still felt "off," but I figured it was because of having a stomach bug and lack of sleep from the week. So I went out for my morning coffee, sat there for a while and then decided afterward I would stop at an urgent care clinic in hopes of getting a prescription that could alleviate my symptoms. Since I had dinner plans that night with friends, as well as plans for the Super Bowl the next day, I was hoping for a quick fix to the problem.

The urgent care clinic ran routine blood tests. Sitting behind that room curtain, I wondered what was taking so long. It had been over an hour. Finally, the doctor arrived; she was just beginning to flip through the blood work results as she walked in. I saw her face change, and she was quiet as she continued to flip through the paperwork. It scared me. She looked up at me and asked, "Did you know you have diabetes?" I looked at her like she was dead nuts. I thought she was rude and replied,

"I don't *have* diabetes." She said my blood sugar levels were dangerously high, and that I would need to be taken to an emergency room right away. Being flippant, I said, "Look. I just drank a large, sugary coffee beverage and a bowl of oatmeal. *Of course* my sugar levels are going to be a little high."

I ended up going to the emergency room solely to appease them and have them realize they had made a big mistake. I didn't call anyone, or even cancel my dinner plans with my friends, because I figured the situation would be resolved before then.

It was there that I was initially diagnosed with type 2 diabetes and mild DKA [diabetic ketoacidosis] by the emergency room physician. Once I was checked in to the hospital, the rounding endocrinologist re-evaluated the diagnosis. I was 106 pounds and 5'6". He gathered more blood work and sent it to the lab, which confirmed I had type 1 diabetes. He said it was rare for someone in their 30s to be diagnosed with type 1. Like most other newly diagnosed diabetics will probably tell you, it changed my life forever.

Tell me about your celiac diagnosis. It came five months after your diabetes diagnosis, that must have been completely overwhelming. How did you cope with the emotional side of a dual diagnosis?

Overwhelming is a good word, but doesn't begin to describe how I felt when I was diagnosed with celiac disease. There's a little bit of a back-story.

My celiac diagnosis was in July 2010, but three months prior I had been diagnosed with another auto-immune disease, Grave's disease. In May 2010, I underwent radioactive iodine therapy to treat the Grave's disease. The treatment consisted of receiving radiation orally by swallowing it. It was delivered to me each day in the hospital by a man in a hazmat suit, and I wondered why I wasn't in a hazmat suit, too. He told me "Don't let this sit in your mouth for any period of time. You have to swallow it immediately or the wrong part of your body could absorb the radiation." Scary! That treatment went on for about a week. I was considered radioactive for a period of time afterwards, so no one was allowed to come around me. I was still very ill with the new diabetes diagnosis, but was stuck taking care of myself since no one could come over.

By July, I was still feeling very sick. I didn't know if it was from the Grave's disease or the diabetes. I had diarrhea, the kind that makes you afraid to stand up at work out of fear of having an accident. I began to bring an extra pair of under-pants to work "just in case." Then came the onset of constipa-tion and severe bloating. Really, really bad bloating. I couldn't put pants on and so I purchased a bunch of cheap summer dresses I could wear to work. I couldn't stand any pressure on my stomach at all, it was so painful. I was embarrassed because people around me were jokingly telling me I looked like I was nine months pregnant. I writhed around night after night in pain, unable to sleep.

I complained to my endocrinologist about it during a rou-tine A1C check. He ran the blood work to check for additional auto-immune diseases. The blood test came back positive for celiac disease, which was confirmed by an endoscopy two days later. The gastroenterologist left me a voice mail stating I had a "surprisingly bad" case of celiac disease with a large amount of damage to my small intestine. He told me it was one of the worst cases he'd seen. He wouldn't be referring me to a dietitian, the voicemail said, because the feedback he'd been given by his celiac patients was that the dietitian visits were not helpful. He suggested I contact a local celiac support group for further infor-mation, and provided the name of a contact person. That was the end of the voicemail.

I was driving in my car when I listened to the voicemail, and I began crying so hard I had to pull off the road. I was hys-terical. It was the third auto immune disease diagnosis in a five-month period. What was wrong with me? I used to be so healthy. What had I done wrong? Was I going to get another one? When would it stop?

Two medical diets, one life. It certainly wasn't easy. Still fresh off of a type 1 diabetes diagnosis and Grave's disease treatment and then having to learn what a gluten free diet entailed was very difficult. I don't think I could have handled it all emotionally if I hadn't found an outlet, which was to learn as much as I could about my new diseases. I became obsessed, really. I bought EVERY book I could find on diabetes and celiac disease. And the more I read, the more frustrated I became because a gluten-free diet is not necessarily diabetic friendly. I tried to find foods that satisfied the requirements of both diseases, and my options seemed really limited. I really questioned whether or not I was going to be able to manage it.

Did you meet with a nutritionist to get a better understanding of celiac? Do you know why the two diseases are so closely related? Have you met other women with celiac and diabetes?

I did eventually meet with a dietitian, several actually. I found that almost every dietitian I met with did not have a strong working knowledge of the gluten-free diet. They could provide an overview of the diet, but I already knew the overview. I needed details; specifics about what I could eat. Some directed me to eat foods that I later discovered were not gluten free. Another dietitian was looking up information on the internet right alongside me during my appointment, trying to find options. It wasn't until I found a dietitian who specialized in diabetics who have celiac disease that I FINALLY got the answers I needed.

There are links between my three autoimmune diseases. Most of my physicians feel that my diseases were not diagnosed in the order in which I actually got them. I had celiac disease first, that much they know, and from the level of damage to my intestines, it appeared I had it for many years without any symptoms. There isn't a way for them to determine if one disease caused another, but what they do know for sure is that these three diseases are commonly diagnosed in tandem. They "run in the same circles," as my doctor put it, and getting one of them dramatically increases your chances of getting another. Current research estimates that *one in every ten type 1 diabetics has celiac disease*, or will be diagnosed with it in their lifetime, and some physicians in the field are recommending that type 1 diabetics be checked annually.

I felt so alone after my diagnoses. No one understood my new diet (not even me). I felt some friends pull away. It wasn't until I found the diabetes online community that I started to feel hopeful again. I have met a couple of women who have "celiabetes," as one of them calls it! Only they understand how difficult it is to eat outside of the house! But I also enjoy talking with people who have only diabetes or only celiac. I learn so much! It's refreshing to talk to people who *get it.* And it's fun to have our inside jokes that only those with the disease will comprehend.

Tell me about the food you eat. What can you eat? What can't you eat? Do you eat snacks? If so, what? What foods do you miss the most, if any?

Nowadays, I have a really great handle on what I can and cannot eat. I can't eat wheat, barley, rye, malt, or noncertified gluten-free oats, or anything that may have been cross contaminated with them. The cross contamination concern is what makes eating at restaurants difficult. You learn to ask the manager A LOT of questions before eating at their establishment! Many restaurants now have gluten-free menus, but you must be careful. An example is a local pizza restaurant that advertised their new "gluten-free pizzas" in the newspaper. When I called the restaurant to inquire, I found out that they do not have a separate prep area for the gluten-free pizzas, and that the same sauce spoon was used for both pizzas. So literally, the sauce spoon would be used to smear sauce on a regular pizza, and then used on the gluten-free pizza. That's a celiac no-no! It only takes trace amounts of gluten to cause an autoimmune reaction.

I have found some great whole-grain, gluten-free breads, pastas, and crackers that I eat now. And I eat foods I hadn't previously, like quinoa and polenta. These are great foods! Because I am diabetic, I watch the amount of carbs I eat and try to not eat too many high-carb snacks. But when a snack attack hits me, there is no shortage of options! There are a few dedicated gluten-free bakeries where I live, so every once in a while I'll stop and pick up a treat, like a cupcake. But it's not very often because gluten-free items are very expensive. I'd still rather go purchase a single cupcake (or two) from the bakery than make a whole pan of them myself and have them sitting in front of me at home.

The food that I miss the most is fast food. I miss the convenience of being able to run through a drive thru and grabbing a quick bite to eat. I hope that in the future, the fast food chains will create gluten-free menus. I also miss fresh, hot, airy French bread and croissants, and I miss being able to quickly grab a light frozen dinner from the freezer section of a grocery store for two dollars. And I really miss couponing! There are rarely coupons for gluten-free food in the Sunday newspaper.

My favorite recipe is *Crustless Spinach Quiche*. It's both celiac and diabetic friendly, and is so delicious and easy!

Crustless Spinach Quiche

2 teaspoons canola oil
1 medium yellow onion, chopped
1 (10 oz.) pkg frozen, chopped spinach, thawed and drained
1-½ cup reduced fat cheddar, grated
6 large egg whites
1 large egg
1/3 cup nonfat cottage cheese
1/4 teaspoon ground red pepper (cayenne)
1/8 teaspoon salt
1/8 teaspoon nutmeg

Preheat oven to 375. Coat 9-inch pie plate with nonstick cooking spray, set aside. In skillet over medium-high heat, heat oil. Add onion, stirring for 5 minutes or until translucent.

Add spinach and stir until moisture has evaporated, about 3 minutes. Sprinkle cheese evenly in prepared pie plate. Top with spinach mixture. In a medium bowl, whisk together egg whites, egg, cottage cheese, red pepper, salt, and nutmeg. Pour egg mixture evenly over spinach. Bake for 30–40 minutes, or until set. Let stand for 5 minutes, then cut into wedges and serve.

Bon appetit!

Do you feel "high maintenance" when it comes to food? What are the challenges?

Having celiac disease definitely makes me feel high maintenance when it comes to food, but having diabetes doesn't. With diabetes, you can still pretty much eat whatever you want. But having celiac disease makes it challenging to eat outside of your house. Not just at restaurants, but at other people's homes, and at work functions or while traveling. Many people think they understand what's involved in making a gluten-free meal, but unfortunately many don't understand the cross contamination aspect of the diet. There's nothing worse than when a dear friend surprises you with something "gluten free" that they made for you, and you are scared to death to eat it. You don't want to be rude, but you also don't want to risk getting long-term intestinal damage from eating it. To avoid those situations, I usually always bring my own meal if I am invited to eat at someone else's house. Now, I know that's not how all celiacs do it, but that's how I choose to do it. It takes the stress off of the host and then I know that I have a safe meal to eat. My friends have become accustomed to this practice, so it's not a big deal. In addition, I will always bring a gluten free dish I can pass for others to eat.

Grocery shopping can also be a challenge; often I will have to look up items on my phone or call an 800 number to see if the products are gluten free. It can make for some long shopping trips. This way of living becomes a part of your daily life, so you adjust.

What are the positive aspects of these diagnoses, if any? What have you learned?

The only positive aspects of these diseases, in my opinion, are the wonderful people you meet along your journey. I have made new friends through in-person support groups and online communities. But for me, that's it. Having a disease of any kind is never a good thing, and having these two together, in particular, can take a toll on you socially and financially. There is never a day when I wake up happy to have diabetes or celiac disease. But they are a part of my life and I've learned to accept them. They have taught me to protect how I see myself. *Don't see sick. See healthy.* I've learned how to live a happy, grateful life in spite of them.

Claire Blum had diabetes for nearly fifteen years when she first began noticing strange symptoms. "It felt like hypoglycemia within ten to fifteen minutes of some of my meals, when indeed my blood sugar was not low. Sometimes my blood sugar would drop later on, and other times it would climb. When I told my endocrinologist he responded as though it was ridiculous, and I thought better of sharing such unexplainable things. As the years passed I began having unusual periods of shortness of breath, yet pulmonary function and cardiac stress tests showed that I was perfectly healthy. I also had airway spasms as often as two to three times per week, during which my husband would stand by waiting to see if I would pass out, or if I would be able to relax out of the spasm on my own. Even though the spasms were severe, they didn't concern me a great deal because I believed they were caused by a reactive reflex when larger particles of food hit the back of my throat, as a result of structural damage and facial trauma at the time of an earlier automobile accident. As the years passed, however, my health slowly declined, and it became increasingly difficult to make it through the absolute essentials of everyday life. I was frequently overwhelmed, irritable, and edgy, and found it difficult to focus. In time I developed gastrointestinal symptoms, with bloating, burping, stomach pain, and irregular bowel movements that fluctuated between crampy loose stools and small hard balls that were difficult to pass, and my 'hypoglycemic-like' episodes following meals were often incapacitating.

"By this time I had an endocrinologist with whom I was comfortable discussing my symptoms, and even though I showed evidence of delayed gastric emptying, he felt certain that I did not have neurogenic gastroparesis because I do not have symptoms of nerve damage in other parts of my body. I began noticing that my symptoms worsened following meals filled with pasta or breads and other gluten-containing foods, but I was reluctant to test for celiac, because I knew how life changing the diagnosis could be. My endocrinologist agreed that it was possible, but he waited to test until I actually asked, nearly a year later. When the tests came back, everything was negative for celiac, and he advised me that it was safe to continue with my present diet. In the meantime, it had been determined with use of spirometry that my difficulty in breathing was largely due to severe reactivity to particles of latex in the air, even though my blood tests for latex allergy had also come back negative. As I became aware of food sensitivities that are commonly seen in people who have latex allergies, I began eliminating those foods from my diet, and my airway spasms nearly disappeared, but my gastrointestinal symptoms and difficulty in breathing continued, and I still had those "hypoglycemic-like episodes.

"A few years later, I became friends with a dietitian who specialized in food sensitivities and LEAP [lifestyle eating and performance] testing, and she immediately identified my gastrointestinal symptoms and difficulty breathing during the night as likely signs of gluten sensitivity. She told me that gluten sensitivity can move on a continuum of no sensitivity at all, at one end of the scale, to outright celiac on the other. I also learned that the blood tests commonly used to screen for celiac are not specific enough to detect the presence of gluten sensitivity in all individuals. So reluctantly at first, yet feeling I had nothing to lose, I decided it was time for trial of a gluten-free diet. Within a week my symptoms began to subside, gradually at first, and more markedly in the weeks and months to come. My A1C came down from the 7.5 to 8 percent I was struggling to maintain, into the 5.8 to 6.5 percent range. Needless to say my endocrinologist was very impressed and checked my CBC [complete blood count] several times to be certain I was not anemic. He now refers clients who test negative for celiac, but demonstrate remarkable symptoms, to his dietitian for trial of a gluten-free diet.

"In addition to my gluten sensitivity, I later found, with use of LEAP testing, that I was reacting to commonly used food additives and preservatives and several additional foods. With elimination of these 'reactive foods' in my diet, I rarely experience those unexplainable 'hypoglycemic-like' symptoms following my meals, which I now know were indication of adrenalin response to the reactive foods, similar to the adrenalin response seen with hypoglycemia."

I asked Claire about managing her blood glucose levels during this transition and she said that it wasn't easy.

"Sometimes I feel jaded because the elimination of gluten from my diet seems like it would be a 'piece of cake' compared to elimination of the many 'other' foods I've found a need to eliminate. For those with gluten sensitivity alone, there are numerous products and specialized flour mixes, developed by gourmet pastry chefs, that make replacement of gluten-containing foods much easier than it was ten years ago. Mindful attention to my body and the way it responds to the foods that I eat has made this process much easier, and I have learned a great deal about the many hidden ingredients found in prepackaged foods that often contribute to food sensitivities.

"The payoff has been well worth the effort, in that my blood glucose is much easier to control, and I feel so very much better . . . like my body is finally getting the nutrients it had been craving and needing. My thinking is clearer, and I am much less irritable and edgy. I feel like a new person!

"Given the diversity of my food sensitivities the bulk of my diet is whole grain cereals such as millet, corn grits, and buckwheat; whole grain rice and potatoes; lots of veggies; a few fruits; and a diversity of nuts and seeds to balance out the protein in my meals. I have developed recipes for granola that makes an easy 'to go' meal, and shortbread tea cakes that give me a crunchy diversion from the basics!

"I've worked a great deal with my dietitian friends to be certain I am getting adequate protein and nutrients from the foods I am able to eat, but most of my learning has been on my own. I learn best by reading and experimentation that helps me discover what works for my body.

"I miss a lot of the foods I used to be able to eat, but I choose not to spend time thinking about it. I find that 'eating to live' rather than 'living to eat' provides me with so much more energy and life that I wouldn't want to go back to feeling the way I did. In some ways it actually simplifies life, in that I know what I am going to eat and what I need to buy. . . . Traveling is a different story, as I have to carry everything I will need to eat. We don't eat out very often, and if we do, I again carry all my own food. In that regard, it has probably been more difficult for my husband than it has for me, as it has taken some time for us to learn ways of navigating the kitchen to make certain he is able to get a variety of foods that he enjoys."

AUTHENTIC ADVICE

■ *I am a decently educated e-patient so I haven't met with a dietitian or doctor about this. My allergist thinks it's great that I avoid gluten since it bothers me and is glad that I worked to figure out what was bothering—especially since my celiac test came out negative.* ■ Sysy Morales

■ *For weddings or BBQs I either eat before the event, or I bring my own food to eat. I have amassed quite a collection of different sized coolers to fit different situations! And I always have some gluten-free bars stuffed in my purse.* ■ Nikki Coar

(continued)

AUTHENTIC ADVICE (continued)

■ *Don't be afraid of finding out what's going on. Read and learn, explore the possibilities, experiment, and listen to your body. It will tell you what to do! The pain and discomfort of eating foods you are reactive to is a steep price to pay for your health, well-being, and enjoyment of life. Nothing tastes as good, as feeling good feels! LEAP testing may be helpful in deciphering out the variables (www.nowleap.com).* ■ Claire Blum

9   What Do I Eat When I'm Hungry? Snacks

I remember when I was first diagnosed with diabetes sitting on the hospital bed watching the nutritionist play with a plastic piece of chicken, a plastic apple, a plastic slice of bread, and a plastic head of broccoli. She was talking in what sounded like a foreign language about food exchanges, starches, and sliding scales (remember this was 1985). When she started talking about a sliding scale and counting carbohydrates to determine how much insulin I'd need to take thirty minutes before my meals, I zoned out. Done playing with the food, she looked up and asked if I had any questions.

"What do I eat when I'm hungry?" I asked. She looked at me and paused a moment too long.

"Snacks you mean?" she asked. I nodded. I was thinking about my friends who between meals, went to the mini-mart across the street from school (I attended a private boarding school) and bought Sugar Babies to snack on in class. When study hall was over at 9 pm, we could go to the "den" and order fries and a milkshake. I loved the chocolate milkshakes from the den.

"You can have something from the Free Food List like pickles, raw vegetables or nuts," she said, handing me a very short list of Free Foods. A pickle was the last thing I craved when I was hungry. In teenage-like fashion, I tossed the list onto the floor as soon as she left the room.

It's been twenty-six years since that conversation and I am now a mom to three boys. Thankfully, a lot has changed when it comes to a "diabetes diet," and the way I eat is far less restricted than when

I was first diagnosed. Although when it comes to eating between meals, nuts are still my go-to snack! One of the challenges I face when it comes to eating "right" as a mom is that my pantry is filled with all sorts of carb-heavy, processed snacks. We have chips, pretzels, squeezable yogurts, granola bars, fruit snacks, and crackers, and most of the time, I'm the one serving them up. I'm used to saying no to myself and I've been around long enough to know that if I ate one of my son's granola bars, I'd feel like crap. So I don't. Most of the time I'm not even tempted and will reach for a jar of almonds or a slice of cheese, but still. It's harder to say no when my pantry is filled with these snacks. I know what you're thinking: Why don't you give your kid's low-carb snacks? It's a long and complicated answer but the short version is that growing up with vegetarian, hippie parents who were very strict about food has made me want to let my kids snack on what they want to snack on within reason, and that means chips, cookies, and granola bars. They get their fruits and veggies too, but I made the choice to offer freedom when it comes to snacks.

INTRODUCING THE *DIABETES LIFE* HEALTHY, LOW-CARB SNACK LIST!

Snacks can be a double-edged sword for people with diabetes. They may help stave off hunger and overeating, while keeping blood sugar levels from dropping too low. But serious snack attacks can also derail your best efforts to eat healthy and manage your weight. Read on for the best in diabetes-friendly snacking and sweet treats.

Mozzarella String Cheese

This is the new Snickers bar. Talk about a perfect, portable snack. How do you eat your string cheese? Do you peel it carefully with your fingers or your teeth? Or do you just chomp, chomp, chomp until it's gone?

Carbs: Less than 1 gram

Popcorn

Popcorn is a whole grain—did you know that? Popcorn delivers a nice dose of fiber and is a versatile snack. You can stick to butter, sprinkle with grated parmesan or Brewer's yeast, or make a sweet treat by drizzling with sugar-free chocolate syrup.

Carbs: 12 grams in 2 cups

Cottage Cheese and Berries

This will make you feel healthier just by having a dish in front of you. You get all the benefits of dairy protein and fat, plus a good dose of antioxidants. What could be better?

Hint: If cottage cheese has always seemed a little icky to you, try sprinkling cinnamon and sugar substitute on top and sticking it in the oven for a few minutes, berries and all.

Carbs: 15 grams in 1/2 cup cottage cheese and 1/2 cup blueberries

Whole Wheat Crackers and Natural Peanut Butter

This is perfect for a salty, crunchy fix. Plus, you get protein, fiber, and good-for-you unsaturated fats.

Carbs: 15 grams in 3 Triscuits with 2 tablespoons peanut butter

Hard Boiled Egg

The incredible edible is truly a perfect food—with a nutrient list that reads like the side of a multivitamin label. It's also oh-so-satisfying.

Carbs: Less than 1 gram (and more than 6 grams of protein!)

Edamame (a.k.a., Green Soybeans)

Edamame are a diabetes super-snack. Buy them frozen in the pod, boil for five minutes, and voila! Pick up the pods and suck out the tender beans.

Carbs: 15 grams per cup (and 8 grams of fiber!)

A Pear (With a Handful of Almonds)

This has the added snack benefit of slowing you down a bit. It's hard to inhale a fruit you have to take bites of while navigating around seeds and a stem. And although they're easy to overeat, nuts have to be chewed pretty thoroughly. Eat your almonds one at a time, chew slowly, and savor their buttery goodness.

Carbs: 16 grams in a small Asian pear and 12 almonds

Sugar-Free Jello

This is arguably the most satisfying zero-carb sweet treat out there. Although it may not win in the nutrients contest, it can at least do a good job making your nails stronger.

Carbs: 4 grams in a cup of sugar-free Jello with 4 tablespoons whipped topping

Hummus and Veggies

This is the healthy replacement these days for potato chips and sour cream dip. Hummus, a Middle Eastern puree, is made from chickpeas (a.k.a. garbanzo beans) and garlic. It's high in protein and fiber and many other nutrients and, without a doubt, classifies as a diabetes superfood. Add some carrots and celery for dipping, and you know you're doing a good thing for your body.

Carbs: 15 grams in 5 tablespoons of hummus with 4 baby carrots and 4 small celery stalks

Plain Yogurt

To some, yogurt is a nectar from the gods. To others, it's as gross as curdled milk. If you're in the latter group, why not take baby steps?

First, use plain yogurt to make salad dressings and in baked goods. Eventually, graduate to eating it with sugar substitute and berries or crushed nuts. The health benefits are stellar—from the calcium to the friendly bacteria—so it's worth a bit of effort.

Carbs: 12 grams in 6 ounces of plain yogurt or 8 grams in 8 ounces of plain Greek yogurt

Sugar-Free Pudding

Is one of the more decadent treats available, and with a dollop of whipped cream can stand in for someone's beloved chocolate mousse dessert. Swirl a couple of flavors together for that extra *je ne sais quoi*.

Carbs: 12 grams in 1/2 cup

Dark Chocolate (The Higher the Percentage of Cocoa, the Better)

Dark chocolate has been shown to possibly improve health by way of its plant chemicals. And three dark chocolate truffles will cost you only 15 grams of carbs. However, they also come with 220 calories and 13 grams of saturated fat. By anyone's standards, that's a little over the top.

So take a more moderate approach: Have just one dark chocolate truffle, and enjoy every second of it.

Lesley Hoffman Goldenberg's favorite snacks are: "Chocolate Fiber One bars, low-sugar brown sugar oatmeal, Deli Flat with a slice of cheese, Greek yogurt with blueberries, 2 Clementines, and during the summer in NYC, I'll sometimes treat myself to Pinkberry frozen yogurt. I almost always need a snack with carbs in it because I often eat dinner too late and can't last between lunch and a late dinner."

Alyssa Rosenzweig doesn't follow the three-meals-a-day plan. "I eat a little bit of protein and vegetables every few hours," she says. "If

I go too long without eating and get hungry, then my physical state is stressed and I can feel it." Alyssa snacks on deli meat roll ups, nuts, almonds, cherry tomatoes, celery, Kashi dark cherry bars, and pickles. "I don't look strictly at the carb content," she says. "I look at fat, fiber, protein, and carbs."

Rachel Garlinghouse lost a great deal of weight when she was first diagnosed with type 1 diabetes. "I am almost 5 feet 8 inches tall, and upon diagnosis I weighed 97 pounds. I was told to eat high-calorie meals and snack often. Once I gained weight, I was told to eat three meals and three snacks a day, each containing carbohydrates, plenty of fiber, protein, and healthy fats. I was encouraged by professionals and by diabetes media that artificial sweeteners are fine to consume. However, I think they taste terrible, and I gained too much weight when I baked with sugar substitutes, mostly because, as I learned, people who consume fake sugars usually weigh more than those who don't. The theory is that the body knows when it's being tricked and the person over-consumes other foods causing weight gain to make up for the manipulation. I stopped using all faux sugars in my baking and simply used real sugar in reduced amounts. My baked goods tasted better and my weight dropped.

"I usually eat five times a day. Breakfast, lunch, snack, dinner, dessert with my husband before bed. My afternoon snack is usually a small bowl of Kashi Go Lean Crunch, some fruit, and string cheese, a granola bar (if I'm on the go), and the occasional scone and sugar-free vanilla soy iced latte from Starbucks. I usually do bolus for snacks because my snacks tend to be more than 15 grams of carbs. Though, of course, it depends on my blood sugar."

Asha Brown says her "go-to snacks" are "string cheese, V8, almonds (for when I don't need to cover/bolus) and if I need a little extra to get me through to my next meal, I eat dried fruit, (prunes!), apples or if I really need a mini-meal I eat Larabars and Kind bars. They all vary in protein and carbs, so I carry a variety with me when I'm out during the day. If I don't need extra carbs for a snack, I choose protein or very low carb in order to just keep my energy up. I rarely eat full meals. I tend to eat three small meals throughout the morning, which works very well to keep my blood glucose levels stable and to keep my energy up, and then I have a lunch meal sometime in the afternoon. I eat another small balanced mini meal early evening and then another balanced mini meal with my husband when he comes home from work around 7:00 pm. This eating style is my 'normal.'

"Obviously there are days when there is more of a 'three-meal, two-snacks between' kind of deal, but that's usually when we're traveling or on vacation. In my regular daily life I am very active so I don't want to eat larger meals and deal with covering too much, and taking care of unexpected lows. Though they still happen from time to time!"

AUTHENTIC ADVICE

■ *Remember in the movie* Thelma and Louise *how Geena Davis eats tiny bites of a candy bar out of the fridge, opening and closing the door every time and never actually taking the bar out? And then later when they're on the lam she'll only buy tiny airplane sizes of Jack Daniels, never a full-size bottle? I think that's the best model out there for eating right with diabetes. Not the chocolate and whiskey in particular (although I very much admit to both), but the portions and the timing. The smaller you can go and the more evenly you can spread them out throughout the day, the better your numbers will be. I think our bodies work better that way on other levels as well, or at least mine does. It's nice to never feel starving or engorged. It's good to have both your brain and your guts that steady. It takes some work and some getting used to, but really, you're diabetic.* ■ Ann Rosenquist Fee

10 Eating Right at Different Times of Life: Childhood, Adolescence, and Getting Older

Eating right for people with diabetes will change as our bodies change. What is "right" for us when we are a child or a teenager may not be right when we are in our twenties, when we are pregnant, when we are training for a marathon, when we are having menopause, and when we age. As people with diabetes, we have to always listen and learn from our bodies from one stage of life to the next.

FEEDING YOUR CHILD WITH DIABETES

Karen Hargrave-Nykaza's fourteen-year-old son Joel was diagnosed with type 1 diabetes on October 16, 2003 and she says, "From what I do know about people who develop 'issues' with food, or even eating disorders, they are about control and the need to control. That leads me to the conclusion that the more I restrict something, the more my son will need to struggle to control it. If I want it to be a nonissue, I should not forbid it in the first place. The best way to encourage moderation seems to be to practice it myself, and model good choices as an example for my son. Without limiting someone's access to sweets, we hopefully avoid them having the urge to binge on something when they do have the opportunity to eat it. This is especially true of young adults. Adolescence is a time of rebellion, and I know I do not want to give my son a reason to make food a vehicle for rebellion."

Karen and her husband, Kevin, have done what they can to learn as much as possible, not only about the disease itself and how to manage it, but how to deal with the disease while maintaining a "normal" life for Joel and their whole family. After Joel's diagnosis, Karen began searching without success for the unique information needed by the parent of a child with diabetes. When she didn't find that information, she found her own way through dealing with the school system, kids' birthday parties, finding support as a parent, and educating friends and family members about diabetes. After she had done that, she came to the conclusion that she was the best person to write the book she had searched for and imagined as a parent who had just muddled her way through all those things and more. She decided to offer what she had learned with other parents when she wrote *My Child Has Diabetes*.

Karen's son has a friend with diabetes whose mother has been very restrictive with food. "If she wants something sweet, she can't have it. This has created a secretive dynamic between them and in my estimation, an unhealthy relationship with food. When she does have the opportunity to eat sweets, she is less able to regulate herself and make healthy choices because she may only have the chance to eat candy once a month, compared to my son who could eat a small amount of candy every day if he wanted to. It is well documented that teens with controlling parents are more likely to develop eating disorders."

Karen says there is a very fine line between how much control is reasonable, and how much will create a problem for a particular child (or adult). "From the beginning of my son's journey with diabetes, we wanted to create an environment where he was the one making the choices, since it was his life we were affecting. In two more years when our son leaves for college, we will not be there to make choices for him regarding what he eats and how much alcohol he drinks. We have to trust him now to begin making those choices independently."

Q&A WITH KAREN HARGRAVE-NYKAZA

You talk about how restricting food only makes you want them more, and as someone who has lived with the restrictions of diabetes for twenty-six years, I agree! Can you offer any specific anecdotes about how this approach has helped your son have an easier relationship with food?

The best anecdote I can offer in relation to "forbidden foods" is one that has to do with the day my son came home in tears with a donut hole wrapped in a napkin. His over-the-top school nurse wouldn't allow him to eat the treat that everyone else had as part of the class party that day. She felt it was better to make her job easier by making sure he didn't eat the donuts and have his blood sugar go up than to allow him to fit in with his peers by eating what everyone else was eating, and would not have hurt him. She had a real, "not on my watch" attitude when it came to sweets. She would frequently tell my son that if I let him eat this way at home, that was up to me, but when he was at school, she wanted his blood sugar to be "normal." Imagine what my son's relationship with food would be today if the past eight years had been spent living with the restrictions this school nurse tried to enforce. I feel that he would be a binge eater for sure, among other things. Joel has had the same access to sweets that the rest of our family has, and he probably eats the fewest sweets of any of us, by his own choice. I can only imagine the resentment he would have toward diabetes if he felt it ran his life any more than absolutely necessary. There are really no foods that he "can't" eat, and I think that is a much healthier approach. I do see that the attitudes toward food seem to be different for boys and girls, as well as the forbidden aspects of those foods, because girls seem far more concerned with calories and body image than boys, but not always. Joel has even commented on his female peers going high more often because they don't want to wear their pumps and because they can't hide it in their "skinny" jeans—not really a problem that boys are plagued by.

What advice would you offer parents of adolescents with type 1 diabetes in terms of "eating right?"

If a parent of a type 1 diabetic asked my advice about encouraging their adolescent to eat right, I think much more of my focus would be on balance and moderation than calories, carbs, and nutrition. Even though the end result and goals might be the same, I have found that when there is too much emphasis placed on carbs and constantly counting, the pressure can become too much too fast. When an adolescent or their family feels overwhelmed, they can be tempted to just give up and eat whatever they want. Teens who feel that they have a chance at making a difference toward doing what is good for them are a lot more likely to make an effort. Diabetes and eating right needs to be a PART of their life, not define their whole life. Again, if the latter happens, they are likely to be so overwhelmed that they rebel and give up. In our house, we don't have separate rules or guidelines for eating right for our son with diabetes. We all have the same limits. If the rule is one dessert or treat—that is the rule we all follow. If we are splurging on a bigger treat if we eat out, Joel gets to have one, too. Anything that places additional restrictions on him is out in our house.

Talking to Karen made me realize how much easier it is for me, as a forty-one-year-old mom, to live with diabetes than it was when I was a teenager. Kids thrive on routine and during the school years our lives are pretty tightly scheduled. We eat breakfast, lunch, and dinner at the same time almost every day and never go anywhere without a backpack of snacks. (I learned that the hard and expensive way with having to buy expensive snacks at the movie theater, baseball game, or mall.) My fridge is always full of our favorite things. This is completely different than what my life was like when I was a college student at the University of Colorado.

Without a car of my own (until senior year anyway), I was dependant on my friends to take me to the grocery store or the restaurants, bars, and pizza joints off campus when I was hungry. I was a vegetarian (long story) during college, and ate mostly inexpensive, high-carb foods like bagels, pizza, and cereal. I also stayed up late, exercised inconsistently, and as a result, spent a lot of time with high blood sugars. Trying to balance my social life, studies, a part-time job, and my diabetes was a challenge that I wouldn't want to repeat.

Ana Morales, co-founder of *The Girl's Guide to Diabetes* blog, agrees that college is a tough time to balance blood sugars. Diagnosed at three years old, Ana attends college in Virginia. Her post "Diabetes and Food:A University Perspective," discusses some of the challenges of diabetes at college. She says, "One of the first difficulties I encountered as a freshman was figuring out when to eat so that I could maintain some kind of schedule every day. Often times I've had to skip meals or eat a snack instead of something more substantial. This semester, there have been several days where I was in the art studio from 8:30 in the morning to almost 7:00 at night. I tried to pack food, but that was another issue in itself. It's hard to buy food for just myself and not end up wasting any of it. Sometimes I'd bring bags of salad, but they'd freeze if I put them too close to the freezer section of my mini-fridge. Either that or I wouldn't be able to fit them in the fridge at all. I'd buy packs of cheese and turkey and end up having to throw away the last few pieces.

"When I first came to James Madison University, I also discovered that there's lots of salt in the prepared food. Every time I tried to eat grilled chicken or turkey, I couldn't stomach it because of the saltiness. The soups were usually very salty as well. Since my first year, I've found out which places offer better food choices and I just stick to those now."

Eating During Adolescence

Since I wrote my book, *The Smart Woman's Guide to Diabetes*, I've met many moms who ask if my book will help their teenage daughters. I always tell these moms, and their daughters, that I think the teen years are some of the hardest. When I look back at the angry, rebellious girl I was when I was a teenager, I'm amazed by how much my life has changed. I think people in the health care professions and parents need to realize that when you're teaching people "how to eat right with diabetes," it's a different story for teenagers. What works for someone at forty-five years old (maybe a low-carb, fruit and veggie kind of meal plan) probably will not work for a sixteen-year-old girl who wants to eat what her friends are eating. I think eating right is different at every stage of life. So, what do you recommend for adolescents and/or people at varying stages of life when it comes to eating right with diabetes? How can health care professionals customize healthy eating for different stages of life?

Susan Weiner agrees and says teenagers can be challenging on many levels. "When I work with teenagers who are 'angry' about having to deal with their diabetes, I spend a lot of time 'listening' to them. NEVER bark diet orders at a teenager. At first, they might not share any information. Teenagers answer questions with one word answers. I recommend asking why they are in your office. Often the answer is 'because my parents made me come here.' That is an honest response, which should be acknowledged. I ask open-ended questions, which require more than a one word response. Additionally, I focus on the person, not the diabetes. What is important to the teenager? Perhaps they are concerned about their skin, for example. That is a great way to open a discussion about eating more vegetables, which are high in vitamin A. Are they concerned about recent weight gain? Or not feeling comfortable driving because of low blood sugars? Take what's important, and start to make suggestions. Be friendly, and NEVER judge anyone. Having diabetes is hard. Having diabetes and being a teenager is very stressful."

In their 2002 position statement, the American Diabetes Association recommends the following dietary guidelines for childhood, adolescence, and the aging population. They state:

Historically, nutrition recommendations for diabetes and related complications were based on scientific knowledge, clinical experience, and expert consensus; however, it was often difficult to discern the level of evidence used to construct the recommendations. To address this problem, the 2002 technical review and this position statement provide principles and recommendations classified according to the level of evidence available using the American Diabetes Association evidence grading system. However, the best available evidence must still take into account individual circumstances, preferences, and cultural and ethnic preferences, and the person with diabetes should be involved in the decision-making process. The goal of evidence-based recommendations is to improve diabetes care by increasing the awareness of clinicians and persons with diabetes about beneficial nutrition therapies.

Because of the complexity of nutrition issues, it is recommended that a registered dietitian, knowledgeable and skilled in implementing nutrition therapy into diabetes management and education, be the team member providing medical nutrition therapy. However, it is essential that all team members be knowledgeable about nutrition therapy and supportive of the person with diabetes who needs to make lifestyle changes.

Nutrition Recommendations for Children and Adolescents

Nutrition recommendations for children and adolescents with type 1 diabetes should focus on achieving blood glucose goals that maintain normal growth and development without excessive hypoglycemia. This can be accomplished through individualized food and meal planning, flexible insulin regimens and algorithms, self blood-glucose monitoring, and educa-tion-promoting decision making based on outcomes.

Nutrient requirements for children and adolescents with type 1 or type 2 diabetes appear to be similar to other same-age children and adolescents. Careful consideration of a child's appetite must be used when determining energy requirements. The ideal method for estimating a child's or adolescent's energy needs is a food/nutrition history of a typical daily intake, providing that growth and development are within normal limits. An evaluation of weight gain and growth begins at diagnosis by recording height and weight on pediatric growth charts. Adequacy of energy intake can be evaluated by following weight gain and growth patterns on a regular basis.

Withholding food or having a child eat consistently without an appetite for food in an effort to control blood glucose should be discouraged. Macronutrient composi-tion of the nutrition prescription should be individual-ized according to blood glucose and plasma lipid goals and requirements for growth and development.

Nutrition recommendations for youth with type 2 dia-betes focus on treatment goals to normalize glycemia and facilitate a healthy lifestyle. Successful treatment with nutrition therapy and physical activity can be defined as cessation of excessive weight gain with nor-mal linear growth and achievement of blood glucose goals. Nutrition recommendations should also address associated cardiovascular risk factors such as hypertension and dyslipidemia. Behavior modifica-tion strategies to decrease high-energy high-fat food intake while encouraging healthy eating habits and regular physical activity for the entire family should be considered.

Individualized food/meal plans and intensive insulin regimens can provide flexibility for children and adolescents with diabetes to accommodate irregular meal times and schedules, varying appetite, and varying activity levels.

RECOMMENDATIONS

- Individualized food/meal plans and intensive insulin regimens can provide flexibility for children and adolescents with diabetes to accommodate irregular meal times and schedules, varying appetite, and varying activity levels.
- Nutrient requirements for children and adolescents with type 1 or type 2 diabetes appear to be similar to other same-age children and adolescents.

Caroline Hill was diagnosed July 11, 2011 with an A1C of 14.9. "I was eleven years old and had lost twenty-five pounds that summer, but didn't realize it was that much. I still did all my actives like cheer, swim, tumbling, tennis, and/or running, but I was extremely tired. I just thought it was because it was the 100 degree Louisiana weather. I also was very thirsty and had been getting up at night to use the bathroom. That morning I was supposed to be going to church camp, but I was told I needed to get my physical done. At the doctor's office we were told I had type 1 diabetes. I later realized my mom knew I had diabetes after smelling the fruitiness in my breath that morning, but at the time I was more worried about missing camp than having diabetes.

"I got a pump (animas ping) the next month and entered junior high (seventh grade) with a new diagnosis that changed my life.

"I handled the diagnosis better than my parents because they knew I had to do it for the rest of my life. It really had not sunk in with me until a male nurse gave me my first insulin shot in my arm, and I cried. From then on, I gave my shots—or my mom, who is a nurse practitioner.

"My family is very supportive and so are my friends except for a few who don't understand diabetes and who make annoying comments that I CAN'T eat foods like pizza. I realize it might not be the best choice, but on special occasions I do eat pizza. Ignorance can get on my nerves, but I've learned to ignore it."

Caroline met with a nutritionist in the hospital when she was diagnosed, and continues to meet with the nutritionist during doctor appointments, and says she learns a lot each time. "It's good to have a refresher. At first I ate only healthy foods, then I started sliding and eating more like a normal kid, but overall I eat healthy, check my blood sugar, calculate my carbs and take insulin. I don't eat candy (unless I'm low) or drink cokes/Dr. Peppers, but I don't miss them. I think I do eat healthier now, and even my friends will make healthier choices when with me. My biggest food problem is grazing (like at a party) or because I'm bored. I don't tend to feel frustrated with having to count carbs, especially with the apps on my phone."

Caroline's mom Ashlea says their life changed when Caroline was diagnosed. "I started reading every label before it went in my buggy. I now look for lowest carbs instead of just lowest price. I try to cook more balanced and include all food groups and try and stay away from processed foods. I made very few foods off limits (except for regular soft drinks and real syrup), and if she wants a certain food, she eats it, but we do eat healthier. With four children we have busy schedules, so we still eat out a lot but try to eat balanced. We've learned the foods that elevate her BG and try to avoid them during evening meals. Guacamole is one of her favorite foods, but it drives her BG up like crazy no matter how much we bolus or extend it out. So we make it a special food. I no longer buy Pop Tarts or sugary cereals, so it's easy for her to make good choices because we didn't need those foods either.

"I made the entire family eat healthy and have explained to them the benefits of why we have done this. At times it is more difficult to control her food choices because she wants to be 'normal' and eat whatever she wants whenever she wants, and she needs to be reminded then of better food choices. I am the one who stays up late checking her BG and bolusing for her. Overall the teenage stage hasn't been difficult because Caroline is very compliant. Since I do this for my 'paid job' then with her at home, I'm reading and studying the disease; it interests Caroline, too. She has said since she was a small child that she wanted to be a doctor, and diabetes has opened her eyes to endocrinology."

Eating in the Middle

The American Diabetes Association's nutrition recommendations for "specific populations" includes: people with type 1 diabetes, people with type 2, and pregnant or nursing moms. They state that those of us "in the middle" (not children, the elderly, pregnant women and/or people suffering from complications) should follow the good old-fashioned insulin-to-carb calculations.

Per the American Diabetes Association: "The first nutrition priority for individuals requiring insulin therapy is to integrate an insulin regimen into their lifestyle. With the many insulin options now available, an appropriate insulin regimen can usually be developed to conform to an individual's preferred meal routine, food choices, and physical activity pattern. For individuals receiving basal-bolus insulin therapy, the total carbohydrate content of meals and snacks is the major determinant of bolus insulin doses. Insulin-to-carbohydrate ratios can be used to adjust mealtime insulin doses. Several methods can be used to estimate the nutrient content of meals, including carbohydrate counting, the exchange system, and *experience-based estimation.*" That's my favorite line right there: "experience-based estimation," because that is how I live my life. I have never been good at math and it seemed like a cruel fate that with my diabetes diagnosis, I would have to spend my life (and every meal) struggling to make calculations. My math skills have never improved and that's why I continue to follow the "experience-based estimation" method. It made me feel better to discover that my method actually had a scientific label. I think I can safely assume that with this label, I'm not the only one out there estimating.

- For individuals with type 1 diabetes, insulin therapy should be integrated into an individual's dietary and physical activity pattern.
- Individuals using rapid-acting insulin by injection or an insulin pump should adjust the meal and snack insulin doses based on the carbohydrate content of the meals and snacks.
- For individuals using fixed daily insulin doses, carbohydrate intake on a day-to-day basis should be kept consistent with respect to time and amount.
- For planned exercise, insulin doses can be adjusted. For unplanned exercise, extra carbohydrate may be needed.

Lelsey Hoffman Goldenberg says she eats much differently than when she was younger. "First of all, I eat more consistently—I eat at similar times on most days and similar enough kinds of foods. I find that staying consistent helps maintain and regulate my blood sugars and prevents unnecessary spikes later on. I am more aware than I used to be of calories, fiber content, and carb counting. I also like fruits and vegetables more than I did when I was younger, so I'm more drawn to eating them as snacks. In addition, I can now recognize that after I eat a huge snack of French fries or nachos, for example (which I've probably done once), I emotionally don't feel great so I try to make snack choices that are smart both emotionally, physically and diabetically (is that a word?)."

Rachel Garlinghouse was diagnosed when she was in her mid-twenties and is in her early thirties now, so she says she's "fairly new to diabetes."

"At the beginning of my disease, I concentrated on carb counting. As I pursued learning more about nutrition, I began to look at food as a whole—not just focusing on the carbohydrates. I've learned about the glycemic index, organic foods, vitamin D, fiber, and so much more. I have always loved to bake. When I was first diagnosed I made everything as low sugar as possible by baking with artificial (baking friendly) sweeteners. I found myself rapidly gaining weight, and I couldn't figure out why. Then I learned that faux sugars don't satisfy the body like real sugar does, and people who consume a lot of sugar-free/artificially sweetened foods tend to be heavier. The theory is that they are less satisfied and consume more calories. I believe we are better off eating the real thing: real butter (not hydrogenated-oil laden margarine), real eggs (fat isn't all bad!), real sugar. I've been able to maintain my weight on real foods.

"From the beginning of my diagnosis to now, my eating habits have drastically changed. I eat a mostly organic, mostly vegetarian diet with a lot of raw fruits and veggies. I eat smaller portions, and I'm careful to avoid what I know will spike my sugars. I'm smarter now, healthier now, and happier, too!"

Asha Brown's eating style of mini meals has been pretty consistent throughout her life. "I've been active in dance and theater ever since I was diagnosed (age five), but I used to eat a lot more processed 'healthy' foods that were convenient in college. In the past four years I have chosen to eat more foods that I prepare myself. It takes a little more planning and time commitment but it's worth it to me to trust that the food I am putting into my body is making it happy, healthy, and stronger, instead of loading me up on all the horrible chemicals found in frozen meals and fast food. I have never eaten fast food except for the occasional soft-serve ice cream (my favorite summer treat!)."

Older Adults with Diabetes

When it comes to older adults, the American Diabetes Association says:

There is limited research on changing nutritional needs with aging, and virtually none in subjects with diabetes. Therefore, nutrition recommendations for older adults with diabetes must be extrapolated from what is known from the general population. The most reliable indicator of poor nutritional status in the elderly is probably a change in body weight. In general, involuntary gain or loss of more than ten pounds or 10 percent body weight in less than six months indicates a need to evaluate if the reason is nutrition-related.

The need for weight loss in overweight older adults should be carefully evaluated. Older people with diabetes, especially those in long-term care facilities, tend to be underweight rather than overweight. Low body weight has been associated with greater morbidity and mortality in this age group.

Exercise training can significantly reduce the decline in maximal aerobic capacity (VO₂) that occurs with age, improve risk factors for atherosclerosis, slow the decline in age-related lean body mass, decrease central adiposity, and improve insulin sensitivity; all of which is beneficial for the older adult with diabetes.

A daily multivitamin supplement may be appropriate for older adults, especially those with reduced energy intake. All older adults should be advised to have a calcium intake of at least 1,200 mg daily.

The imposition of dietary restrictions on elderly residents with diabetes in long-term health facilities is not warranted. Malnutrition and dehydration may develop because of lack of food choices, poor quality of food, and unnecessary restrictions. Specialized diabetic diets do not appear to be superior to standard (regular) diets in such settings. Therefore, it is recommended that residents be served the regular (unrestricted) menu with consistency in the amount and timing of carbohydrate. There is no evidence to support diets such as 'no concentrated sweets' or 'no

*sugar added,' which are often served to the elderly in
long-term care facilities. Furthermore, it may often be
preferable to make medication changes to control
blood glucose than to implement food restrictions.*

Camille Baynard Izlar, MS, RD, CDE, BC-ADM, has lived with type 1 diabetes for forty-four years. She is an athlete who has run several marathons and rides horses just about every day and recommends getting out into the world to see what works for you. "Test the waters," she says, "because there is no cook-book answer." Izlar says knowing your body is the key to blood sugar management. "Carbs are not bad for you by any means. We just have to figure out how to take the right amount of insulin." A firm believer in not overtreating lows, she carries Smarties with her when she runs and keeps records of her diet and exercise. A running injury has kept her off the track and she's had to adjust her insulin and diet for horseback riding, which affects her blood sugars differently.

Jeanne Maggiora Hatcher says, "I know more now. Cheetos and orange juice are definite NOs for me. Skim milk is my best friend for lows. I've lived with diabetes for thirty-nine of my forty and one-half years."

The information on eating right with diabetes is vast and constantly seems to be changing. An updated systematic review of the literature on diabetes and food titled *Macronutrients, Food Groups, and Eating Patterns in the Management of Diabetes*, was conducted in 2008 and states:

*The literature on nutrition as it relates to diabetes
management is vast. We undertook the specific topic
of the role of macronutrients, eating patterns, and
individual foods in response to continued controversy over independent contributions of specific
foods and macronutrients, independent of weight
loss, in the management of diabetes. The position of
the American Diabetes Association (ADA) on MNT*

[macronutrients] is that each person with diabetes should receive an individualized eating plan. ADA has received numerous criticisms because it does not recommend one specific mix of macronutrients for everyone with diabetes. The previous literature review conducted by ADA in 2001 supported the idea that there was not one ideal macronutrient distribution for all people with diabetes. This review focuses on literature that has been published since that 2001 date.

I spoke with Stephanie Dunbar, MPH, RD, director of nutrition and medical affairs at the American Diabetes Association, about the systematic review and she said there is no "one size fits all" when it comes to eating right with diabetes.

Dunbar recommends looking at individual needs. "I see our role as trying to guide healthy choices. What works for you as an individual?" she asks. "Is the person with diabetes looking to lose weight? And what about their cultural traditions?" She adds, "No one knows more about your diabetes than you. You have to make your own best choices."

Dunbar says the key for people with type 1 diabetes is matching food to insulin and the key for type 2s is weight management, especially early on, as weight loss lowers insulin resistance.

Steps to eating right with diabetes:

- Weight loss
- Monitor carb intake
- Low saturated fats
- Choose whole grain instead of processed grain-based foods
- Use the "create your plate" guide, which will help keep carb amounts consistent without a lot of label reading
- Eat more nonstarchy vegetables
- Moderate carbs make sense, 45 to 50 percent of total calories
- Choose what works for you!

AUTHENTIC ADVICE

■ *My best advice to a newly diagnosed woman in regard to eating well is that knowledge is power and you are in charge of yourself. Commit to educating yourself on nutrition. Find out where your food is coming from. Know what you are eating. Furthermore, diabetes is 99 percent managed by the patient. The best dietitian, personal trainer, or endocrinologist in the world cannot manage your disease for you. You have to take charge. This is YOUR life; why not live it happy and healthy? You can do it, girl.* ■ Rachel Garlinghouse

■ *Pay attention to how the food you eat actually makes you FEEL. I found it so much easier to trust what my body was telling me after a meal than any diet book or magazine article. As diabetic women, we are already more in tune with our bodies than most people, and I believe we really have an advantage to discover what eating styles and types of foods help us feel our best. Your body knows what it wants if you take the time to really listen to it!* ■ Asha Brown

■ *I recommend paying attention to how you feel as well as your glucometer readings, serum glucose, and A1C. Moderate carb intake works best for me and for many women with diabetes, but some thrive on a very-low-carb diet. Adjust carb intake gradually and assess after each change. Carb levels may need to be adjusted on a day-to-day basis based on your activity level, hormonal changes, and other factors. Stay flexible, and you'll do great!* ■ Franziska Spritzler, RD, CDE

■ *Try to choose foods that you like, that fill you up and that you're excited about to eat as consistently as possible. But don't deprive yourself, and make sure you're splurging once in awhile and trying new and exciting foods, otherwise you'll be resentful of your lifestyle. I would also remember the power of*
(continued)

AUTHENTIC ADVICE (*continued*)

exercising and how if you want to eat a lot without feeling too guilty, exercising can (semi) allow you to do that every so often. If you're feeling out of control with your eating or blood sugars, the best advice is to start writing everything down—it will help you take control, help establish patterns, and help you feel good about what you're doing right ... because we're all doing something right, we just have to be able to recognize it and praise it. ■ Lesley Hoffman Goldenberg

Resources

Amy Campbell is the author of *Staying Healthy with Diabetes: Nutrition and Meal Planning* and a frequent contributor to Diabetes Self-Management and Diabetes & You. She has co-authored several books, including the newly revised *The Joslin Guide to Diabetes* and the American Diabetes Association's *16 Myths of a "Diabetic Diet,"* for which she received a Will Solimene Award of Excellence in Medical Communication and a National Health Information Award in 2000. Amy also developed menus for Fit Not Fat at Forty Plus and co-authored *Eat Carbs, Lose Weight* with fitness expert Denise Austin.

Amy earned a bachelor's degree in nutrition from Simmons College and a master's degree in nutrition education from Boston University. In addition to being a Registered Dietitian, she is a Certified Diabetes Educator and a member of the Academy of Nutrition and Dietetics, the American Diabetes Association, and the American Association of Diabetes Educators. Since 1995, Amy has been Diabetes and Nutrition Educator at Joslin Diabetes Center, where she is responsible for the development, implementation, and evaluation of disease management programs, including clinical guideline and educational material development, and the development, testing, and implementation of disease management applications. She has developed and conducted training sessions for various disease and case management programs and is a frequent presenter at disease management events.

Sheri Colberg-Ochs is an exercise physiologist, author, researcher, and professor of exercise science at Old Dominion University and an adjunct professor of internal medicine at Eastern Virginia Medical School, both located in Norfolk, Virginia. Having earned her undergraduate degree from Stanford University and a Ph.D. from the University of California, Berkeley, she specializes in research in diabetes and exercise. She continues to conduct extensive clinical research in diabetes and exercise with funding from the American Diabetes Association, National Institutes of Health, and others. In addition to her eight books, she has authored more than 250 research and educational articles on exercise and diabetes. Information about her books and articles can be accessed on her official Web site, www.SheriColberg.com.

Megrette Fletcher is a cofounder of The Center for Mindful Eating. She is a co-author of two books, including *Eat What You Love, Love What You Eat with Diabetes* with Michelle May, MD, and *Discover Mindful Eating: A Resource of Handouts for Health Professionals*, with Frederick Burggraf. She is a registered dietitian and certified diabetes educator and provides diabetes education at a diabetes clinic in New Hampshire.

Mary C. Gannon, Ph.D., Director, Metabolic Research Laboratory, Minneapolis VA Health Care System, Professor, Department of Food Science & Nutrition, Associate Professor, Department of Medicine, University of Minnesota.

Steve Parker, M.D., Hospitalist at Desert Vista Medical Associates, author, diabetes blogger.

Franziska Spritzler, RD, CDE, is a registered dietitian and certified diabetes educator who provides individual counseling and teaches group classes at the VA Medical Center in Long Beach,

California. In addition, she maintains a website devoted to low-carbohydrate diets, www.lowcarbdietitian.com.

Susan Weiner is a Registered Dietitian and Certified Diabetes Educator with a successful private practice in New York. Susan is a contributing medical producer for dLife TV and serves as a member of dLife's prestigious medical advisory board. She has been interviewed on TV many times regarding nutrition and diet. Susan is the lead CDE for Diabetessisters, a non profit organization dedicated to the education and empowerment of women with diabetes. Susan is a nutritionist and certified diabetes educator for the diabetes program for TheBestLife.com, a prominent health and weight loss website. She co-authored the "Medical Nutrition Therapy for Anemia" chapter for Krause's *Food and the Nutrition Care Process, 13th Edition*, published August 2011. She is a well respected lecturer for organizations such as the American College of Sports Medicine, and was the official sports nutritionist for the American Diabetes Association Walk America program. She was an adjunct professor of nutrition at Queens College for more than 13 years and taught at the Academy of Applied Personal Training Education at Hofstra University. Susan earned her Master's Degree in Applied Physiology and Nutrition from Columbia University. She is certified in adult weight management through the Academy of Nutrition and Dietetics.

REAL LIFE EXPERTS

Ann Rosenquist Fee writes, sings and wears an OmniPod pump on her inner thigh in Mankato, Minnesota. Online at www .annrosenquistfee.com.

Rachel Garlinghouse is a type I diabetic living in St. Louis. She loves her full life as a wife, mother of two girls, freelance writer, and writing teacher at Southern Illinois University Edwardsville.

She blogs about life as an adoptive mother and shares healthy living tips at www.whitesugarbrownsugar.com

Riva Greenberg has lived successfully with type 1 diabetes for 40 years, since the age of 18, and 10 years ago become a key influencer in the diabetes community for patients and medical professionals. Author of two books, *50 Diabetes Myths That Can Ruin Your Life and the 50 Diabetes Truths That Can Save It* and *The ABC's Of Loving Yourself With Diabetes*, columnist on the Huffington Post, and through her web site, Diabetes Stories, articles, presentations and workshops, Riva is helping patients live an exceptional life, not *despite* having diabetes but *because* of it. She also helps medical professionals work more effectively with patients by better understanding the patient experience. Riva is a peer-mentor with Sanofi's A1C Champion program and a member of the Diabetes Hands Foundation and the American Association of Diabetes Educators.

Sysy Morales is the founder of the diabetes blog, thegirlsguideto diabetes.com. She is a wife and stay-at-home mother of 3 year old twins. Sysy is a certified health coach, a passionate diabetes advocate, a freelance writer, and a public speaker on the subject of health and nutrition, patient empowerment, and diabetes.

WEBSITES

- A Gluten-Free Guide: www.aglutenfreeguide.com
- A Sweet Life, http://asweetlife.org/
- CalorieKing: www.calorieking.com/recipes/advancedsearch.php (Select "diabetes" and "gluten-free" categories.)
- Celiac.com: www.celiac.com
- University of Chicago Celiac Disease Center, www .celiacdisease.net
- The Celiac Disease Resource: www.celiacresource.org

- Celiac Sprue Association: www.csaceliacs.org
- Celiac Sprue Association: www.csaceliacs.org/recipes.php
- Diabetes 123: www.diabetes123.com/recipes/ (Recipes marked "GF" are gluten-free.)
- The Diabetes Daily, http://www.diabetesdaily.com/
- Diabetes Self Management, http://www.diabetesselfmanagement .com/blog/Amy-Campbell/
- Diabetes Sisters, www.diabetessisters.org
- Diabetes and Mindful Eating, www.mindfuleatinganddiabetes.com
- The Center for Mindful Eating, www.tcme.org
- The Girl's Guide to Diabetes, http://thegirlsguidetodiabetes.com/
- We are Diabetes, http://www.wearediabetes.org

Index